FND Stories

of related interest

Breaking Free from Long Covid
Reclaiming Life and the Things That Matter
Dr Lucy Gahan
ISBN 978 1 83997 350 5
eISBN 978 1 83997 351 2

Pulling Through
Help for Families Navigating Life-Changing Illness
Catherine Jessop
ISBN 978 1 78775 372 3
eISBN 978 1 78775 373 0

What I Do to Get Through
How to Run, Swim, Cycle, Sew, or Sing Your Way Through Depression
Edited by Olivia Sagan and James Withey
Foreword by Cathy Rentzenbrink
ISBN 978 1 78775 298 6
eISBN 978 1 78775 299 3

The Ultimate Anxiety Toolkit
25 Tools to Worry Less, Relax More, and Boost Your Self-Esteem
Risa Williams
Illustrated by Jennifer Whitney and Amanda Way
ISBN 978 1 78775 770 7
eISBN 978 1 78775 771 4

FND Stories

Personal and Professional Experiences of Functional Neurological Disorder

Edited by
**GREGG H. RAWLINGS,
MARKUS REUBER, JON STONE
and MAXANNE McCORMICK**

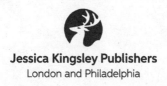

Jessica Kingsley Publishers
London and Philadelphia

First published in Great Britain in 2024 by Jessica Kingsley Publishers
An imprint of John Murray Press

1

The information contained in this book is not intended to replace the services
of trained medical professionals or to be a substitute for medical advice. You
are advised to consult a doctor on any matters relating to your health, and in
particular on any matters that may require diagnosis or medical attention.

Content warning: This book mentions suicide,
suicidal ideation and suicidal thoughts

A CIP catalogue record for this title is available from the
British Library and the Library of Congress
ISBN 978 1 83997 361 1
eISBN 978 1 83997 362 8

Printed and bound in the United States by Integrated Books International

Jessica Kingsley Publishers' policy is to use papers that are natural,
renewable and recyclable products and made from wood grown in
sustainable forests. The logging and manufacturing processes are expected
to conform to the environmental regulations of the country of origin.

Jessica Kingsley Publishers
Carmelite House
50 Victoria Embankment
London EC4Y 0DZ

www.jkp.com

John Murray Press
Part of Hodder & Stoughton Ltd
An Hachette Company

Contents

Acknowledgements

We would like to thank everyone who contributed their story to this book. Unfortunately, we received more contributions than we were able to include, and we are sorry for not being able to include everyone's submission. With their permission, we have acknowledged some of the authors below with their names appearing in alphabetical order. The remaining authors asked to remain anonymous.

Sara Allen
Deborah Anderson
Kelly Anderson
Florencia Austin
Francoise Balfe
Audrey Bart
Teresa Bogner
Melinda Clay-Ota
Jan Coebergh
Conor Coman
Gill Cooke
Emma Coopland-Lee
Jenni Craggs
Siobhan Crombleholme
Kathy Dillon
Paula Gardiner
Chris Gaskell

Cordelia Gray
Catherine Healy
Tami Hennessy
Catherine Hounsome
Luke Hounsome
Allan House
Sarah Hudson
Joyce Love Hurley
Paul Hurlstone
Halimah Hussain
Liliane Huys
Rhiann Johns
Kirsty-Ann Johnstone
Andrew Jones
Anna Jordan
Wesley Kerr
Lorraine King

Emmarae Knight

Sabrina Knott

Katia Lin

Maureen Macdonald

Katie Maciver

Alexandra MacKenzie

Jessica MacKenzie

Anita Mandic

Mary Matthews

Emma McCorkell

Maxanne McCormick

Bianca Millroy

Michelle Montford

Adriana Boschi Moreira

Christine Morrison

Rachel Muir

Anne-Catherine Myriam

Emma Newton

Keira O'Dell

Kim Olsen

David L. Perez

Maria Marta Areco Pico

Hannah Powell

Gregg Harry Rawlings

Markus Reuber

Megan Robertson

Michael Romeo

Shannon Sabiston

Mercedes Sarudiansky

Jacqueline Schofield

Emmi Scott

Charlene Smith

Biba Stanton

Jon Stone

Rachel Thomas

Claire Walton

Toni Warrilow

Rebecca Wright

Teja Zeribi

We also wish to thank Dr Steven Schachter (MD) who created the 'Brainstorms' series, as it was this collection of work that helped inspire the current book. In the 'Brainstorms' series of books, people with lived and professional experience of seizures share their stories with each other and an international readership. Books in this series have been translated into several languages. Two of the 'Brainstorms' books contain stories about functional seizures: *In Our Words: Personal Accounts of Living with Non-Epileptic Seizures* and *Non-Epileptic Seizures in Our Experience: Accounts of Healthcare Professionals*.

Common Acronyms Used

A&E	Accident & Emergency (also known as the Emergency Room (ER))
CBT	Cognitive behavioural therapy
CT	Computerized tomography scan
EEG	Electroencephalogram
EMDR	Eye movement desensitization and reprocessing therapy
FND	Functional neurological disorder
GP	General practitioner (also known as family doctor in some countries)
ICU	Intensive care unit
IV	Intravenous
MRI	Magnetic resonance imaging scan
NEAD, NES or PNES	Non-epileptic attack disorder, non-epileptic seizures or psychogenic non-epileptic seizures (another name for functional/dissociative seizures)
PTSD	Post-traumatic stress disorder
UK	United Kingdom
US	United States

Preface

This book is a collection of stories about FND from the perspectives of people living with the condition, those who support them, and healthcare professionals who care for and treat those impacted by it. Over 70 people from around the world have contributed their stories. Like cameras capturing an object from various directions and with different lenses, these stories provide readers with a multidimensional view of FND. We hope that they will help educate those wanting to learn about the disorder to find out more about the effect it has on people's lives, and increase awareness of the condition. This book should be of interest to anyone who is affected by FND, including people recently diagnosed with the condition, those who have lived with it for some time, their family, friends and support networks, the many different healthcare professionals whose jobs involve caring for this group, commissioners of FND services, and researchers.

An overarching purpose of much of what we do in our professional lives – and of what we ultimately aim to achieve with this book – is to improve the wellbeing of those living with FND, but this book is not intended to act as a guide to treatment or a source of advice. Of course, the accounts of those living with FND and of professionals who reflect on their experiences of providing treatments for people with FND may inspire readers to change their thoughts or behaviours in relation to FND. However, readers will have to extract their learning themselves. As co-editors, we did not want to present didactic lessons. This may seem a more difficult way to challenge previous ways of thinking about the condition, but we think this effort is worthwhile, because it is based on the authentic voices of those with their own lived experience of FND.

FND has been called the most common medical condition that the general public have never heard of. It is estimated that up to 100,000 people in the UK, and up to 500,000 people in the US have FND or FND symptoms. This means that FND is more common than much better-known conditions such as multiple sclerosis or amyotrophic lateral sclerosis (known in the UK as motor neurone disease).

Given how frequent FND is, most healthcare professionals are likely to come across patients with this condition in their working lives and some will encounter patients with FND on an almost daily basis. For instance, some may be surprised to learn that up to one in six people seen in neurology clinics have the condition. But as you will read throughout this book, the symptoms are not always recognized, and FND is under-diagnosed. Many people with the condition experience long delays between the initial development of their symptoms and receiving the diagnosis. Of course, this means the most appropriate treatments are often delayed as well.

In the increasingly sub-specialized world of medicine, the wide range of symptoms which FND can cause means that many different specialists may get involved in the diagnostic process. However, the diagnosis is most likely to be made by experts in neurology and psychiatry. FND is listed in diagnostic classification systems relevant to these specialities (the *Diagnostic and Statistical Manual of Mental Disorders, DSM*, and *International Classification for Diseases, ICD*). These are used by healthcare professionals around the world. Although the *DSM* and *ICD* were created in the 20th century, symptoms which would now be understood as those associated with FND have been described for thousands of years. Throughout this time, FND has been given many different names, such as conversion disorder, 'psychogenic' or 'non-organic' neurological symptoms and, in the 19th century, hysteria. Most of these terms are unhelpful, potentially damaging, and pejorative from today's point of view. While the international classifications aim to standardize the names we should use to avoid confusion, many older and less formal names are still in use. Therefore, in this book capturing the experiences of different individuals, we felt that it was important to allow contributors to use their own terms for their condition if possible.

Some people with FND have a single functional neurological symptom, others experience several symptoms, or their symptoms change and develop over time. Common symptoms experienced as part of FND include seizures, limb weakness, involuntary movements like tremor or spasms (also referred to as dystonia), sensory symptoms and problems with memory and concentration.

Seizures characterized by impaired awareness and self-control are one of the commonest symptoms of FND. Such seizures – which can look and feel like those seen in epilepsy or faints (or syncope) – have also been given many different names over the years (including functional or dissociative seizures, NEAD and PNES). In functional seizures, the brain is in a transient and trance-like state sometimes referred to as 'dissociation'. This is different from epileptic seizures, which are caused by abnormal electrical activity in the brain, or from fainting (syncope) which occurs when the blood supply to the brain is temporarily reduced. Along with epilepsy and syncope, functional seizures are one of the three most frequent causes of transient impairment of consciousness.

Functional limb weakness or movement disorders are other common types of FND. The individual's limb(s) may be paralyzed or heavy, or FND may cause tremor, abnormal gait, and muscle spasms. The symptoms can look and feel like those of Parkinson's disease, multiple sclerosis or stroke.

In functional sensory disorders, people experience changes in normal sensations. They may notice strange sensations, numbness, impaired vision or hearing. Problems with their sense of balance are particularly common. People with persistent dizziness, usually after a dizziness trigger like a bang on the head, may be diagnosed with persistent postural perceptual dizziness (PPPD), which is often considered a subtype of FND.

Cognitive symptoms, like forgetfulness, 'brain fog', and difficulty reading, can also be included in the category of FND. People with functional cognitive disorder will experience difficulties with their thought processes, such as problems with their memory, attention and concentration. People with this disorder may worry they have developed dementia, but unlike people with dementia, those with functional cognitive disorder can usually remember times when they forgot things.

In the past, neurologists tended to diagnose FND by exclusion, doing brain scans and electrical tests like EEG which typically are normal in FND. In the last 20 years, it has become clear that FND should not be diagnosed like that. Instead, people with FND have typical features on clinical assessment such as Hoover's sign of functional leg weakness, the tremor entrainment sign of functional tremor or typical features of a functional seizure. These features mean that the diagnosis of FND is now based on well-described clinical criteria. However, neurological investigations like those mentioned above are still important to see if someone with FND has another neurological condition like epilepsy or stroke *as well*.

One way of understanding FND is to think of your brain as a computer. Of course, our brains are much more sophisticated than a computer, but it is a useful comparison. In someone with FND, the hardware (the physical parts of the computer; the things you can see inside the computer box) is okay, but the software (the programs that run on the computer) is not. For instance, the program for how to walk or talk may not be working as it should be. In someone with functional limb weakness, this means that the signals in the brain are not being produced as they should, or they are interrupted or distorted and never reach the muscles as intended. In a person with functional seizures, awareness of their surroundings may be lost when something goes wrong as the brain is triggered from its resting to a fight or flight state. Like a computer, it may then 'freeze' and have to reboot. If you have ever been working on your computer and the system crashes, perhaps because you had too many 'windows' open or had run out of capacity, then you will know that you first notice that there is a problem on your monitor. However, the monitor is not the cause of the problem.

It is important to stress that FND symptoms are not produced intentionally or self-inflicted, nor is the individual pretending to have an illness or faking or feigning it. To go back to the computer analogy: the fact that a close inspection of the computer which has 'frozen' is unlikely to reveal any snapped wires or damaged electrical components does not mean that the problem which caused the computer to stop working was 'not real'.

As with any other medical condition, it is recognized that a range of different factors can contribute to the development of FND: these include biological (i.e., genetics, hormones, physical injury or infection), psychological (i.e., mental health, thoughts, emotions and behaviours) and social (i.e., stress, relationship, adverse experiences and environment) factors. Within this model, it is possible to identify risk factors that help to explain why some people are more likely to develop FND than others. Such factors may include adverse experiences in the past or present that can be physical, emotional or sexual in nature; or they may be experiences such as those caused by epilepsy, chronic pain or an infection. These are known predisposing factors.

In addition to these risks which individuals may have carried for several years, many people with FND can identify factors that might help to explain why their symptoms started at a particular time (sometimes called precipitating factors). This could be an experience like a migraine aura, a panic attack or a physical injury which created the abnormal 'software' problem in the brain related to a particular body part or experience (such as having a blackout). Once FND has started, many issues may act to maintain the condition and turn it into a more chronic problem (called perpetuating factors), which can involve interactions with healthcare systems that may fail to recognize and help treat the condition.

The most appropriate treatment for FND will depend on the particular symptoms a person is experiencing, but is broadly about 'retraining the brain' with different types of rehabilitation or therapy. These may include psychological therapy, physiotherapy, speech therapy and occupational therapy. Given that some individuals may have been wrongly diagnosed with other medical problems before receiving an accurate diagnosis of FND, optimal treatment may also involve stopping medicines and procedures, as well as managing common co-existing issues like pain, fatigue, low mood or anxiety.

There has been a marked increase over the last 10–15 years in research establishing an evidence base for FND treatments. Research involving functional MRI scans has been particularly helpful to show which brain networks go wrong and contribute to people's FND symptoms. Although functional MRI scans can, so far, not be used to diagnose FND, this research has essentially helped to map out the 'software' problems that are clinically evident in individuals with this condition.

Given the nature of FND and the organization of healthcare services, the condition often falls between treatment pathways and specialities. This means that people with FND may receive treatment advice from a range of health and social care professionals, including, neurologists, psychiatrists, physiotherapists, speech and language therapists, occupational therapists, psychologists, psychological therapists and counsellors, GPs, nurses, emergency care staff, epileptologists, social workers and support workers (this is not an exhaustive list). While people with FND in many countries still struggle to access appropriate treatments, significant progress with the provision of treatment has been made over the last decade. Family and friends can also be a great help for people with FND (which is one of the reasons why we have included their stories in this book). What is more, there are a growing number of third sector and charity organizations aiming to help people with FND – some of these organizations have been listed at the end of this book, under *Helpful Resources*.

In this book, FND emerges as a highly diverse and variable condition which can affect people in many different ways. For example, one person may only experience their FND symptoms occasionally, while another will experience them daily. Some people recover very quickly from FND, but for others the condition becomes more chronic and long term. People can go for long periods without experiencing symptoms before having recurrent flare-ups. There is less variation, however, on how FND impacts people, their families and friends. As mirrored by many research studies, the stories in this book illustrate the various ways in which FND can have a detrimental effect on the quality of life of those affected, and how FND can often, but not always, be complicated by other medical or mental health difficulties, such as depression and anxiety. The stories show us how FND can affect aspects of daily life, including relationships, sleep, work and social and financial matters.

One important way in which people understand, process and make sense of illness is through creating a narrative and telling their story. Just think about the last time you felt unwell and went to your GP, opened up to a friend or family member about how you were feeling, or informed your manager that you did not feel well enough to be at work. In all these circumstances, you will have framed your experience of illness in a story. The stories that we tell of our illnesses often include a beginning (I was feeling well), middle (I became unwell) and ending (I got better). However, when people are living with a medical condition for a long time, when it cannot be cured or if there is uncertainty about how the condition will change or develop, there may not be an ending where someone's health returns to the same level as before. In such cases, the process of storytelling can be even more important, as it can help people to gain a better understanding of the challenges associated with their illness. In fact, there is a lot of research demonstrating how sharing stories of our suffering can be a therapeutic experience.

Sharing personal experiences is likely to be particularly important for a disorder such as FND, in which those affected often feel isolated and do not know anyone else with the condition. Learning of other people's FND stories may help those with the disorder to feel less isolated, validate their own experiences, promote understanding and inspire different ways of coping, or even recovery. The collection of these stories may also help people to overcome some of the stigma and shame often associated with FND. It is no surprise that psychological treatments that are delivered in a group can be effective and, in some cases, are associated with benefits that may not be experienced in treatments provided on an individual basis. There is something powerful about meeting someone who you can identify with because of a shared experience.

To collect the stories for this book, we invited people who use third sector and charity organizations for FND. We also reached out to people who we thought may want to contribute personal or professional accounts of their experiences with the condition online and in person. We encouraged authors to share their stories in any form they wish, including prose, poems, artwork and photographs. To make it easier for contributors to be as open and honest about their experiences and their feelings, and to protect their anonymity, we have pseudonymized all contributions. This means that we have removed or changed information that may identify people, such as names, dates and locations. Where healthcare professionals have written about their experiences or reflections of working with an individual with FND, we have sought reassurance that they have obtained the person's consent for their story to be reflected in their contributions and/or have changed or omitted any identifiable information in a manner that is in line with guidance and policy associated with their profession and employer. The language of the contributions has only been edited lightly by the editorial team, with the hope that we have been able to retain the genuine voice of the author. To that end, we have shared our proposed edits and sought the authors' agreement with our changes, where possible. While we suggested some ideas for aspects of their experiences which people might want to write about, we made it clear that it was most important to us that authors should write about what is most relevant to them. We also want to note that some of the titles of chapters have been proposed by the editors. The aim of this was to help readers in navigating the book as the title will provide some information on the themes and content of each chapter. We hope that the contributors are happy with our suggested titles.

Considerable progress has been made in recent years in terms of how FND is viewed, diagnosed, treated and researched, but the testimonies of the people who contributed to the current book demonstrate that there is still much work to do. We hope that this collection of personal stories will accelerate and shape this process. We are humbled by the response to our call for contributions and very grateful to the authors who have shared their memories, thoughts and feelings so generously. Much like a choir enhances the voice of a single singer, the individual voices emerging from the stories resonate with each other and provide invaluable insight into FND. It has been our privilege to bear witness to the struggles, challenges, tribulations and triumphs of those who have shared their stories with us.

Gregg H. Rawlings,
Markus Reuber,
Jon Stone
and Maxanne McCormick

A Teen's Journey from Functional Seizures to Success

Female, 18 years old, US

FUNCTIONAL SEIZURES

It was nearly time for my parents to switch places visiting me at our local children's hospital. I was 17 and I had been in the hospital for about a week due to complications with my medications. The good news was that I would be heading home tomorrow, yet something didn't feel right: I was nauseous, dizzy, and I just felt out of it.

When my dad came in, I realized I couldn't lift my eyelids or say hello. He greeted me with, 'Hi, excited to go home?' I desperately tried to force my body to snap out of it. I could hear everything around me: my dad settling in for the night, unpacking his stuff, the monitors of patients in other rooms, but I was somehow removed from it. I couldn't move my body.

My dad sat on the bed next to me and asked, 'Have you had dinner yet?' His voice felt miles away. I wanted to respond, more than anything. He said my name, sounding concerned. 'Can you hear me?' I was desperately trying not to scare him, but I couldn't respond.

I could hear him running to get a nurse. The nurse, my favourite from my weeklong stay, was barely in the room for 30 seconds before she shouted, 'Call a code blue!' Panic seared through my body. Code blue? No, I could hear everything! I was here! I was trapped. I heard overhead, 'Code blue...' Suddenly, doctors, nurses and other medical professionals came sprinting into my room and chaos ensued. Half of the team focused on me: what were my vitals? Were my pupils reactive? They opened my eyelids and I heard a nurse say, 'She's got nystagmus.' What did that mean? The other half of the code blue team focused on my nurse and Dad, 'What was she admitted for? What is her baseline mental status?'

The attending doctor who had been treating me took over. He asked, 'Do you know where you are?' Yes. In the children's hospital. But nothing came out except 'hajdjfkfja' in a barely audible whisper. 'Let's get a glucose level on her,' I heard him say. I felt a poke. It didn't hurt. I couldn't feel anything. My dad, his voice hoarse with panic, noted, 'She didn't even flinch. What's happening?' The attending agreed, 'This is completely different from her baseline. She's usually super talkative and working on schoolwork. Call a rapid response team code. Let's get a head CT scan. Call the paediatric ICU and tell them we need a bed stat.' Somewhere in the chaos, I heard, 'Out of the way! I'm her mother, let me see her!' Both of my parents were sobbing and I wanted to reassure them. But I couldn't.

Soon I was being suspended in the air on a sheet, and moved to the CT board. Not for the first time that horrible night, my body betrayed me. I began to seize uncontrollably. My tongue was bleeding. I could hear voices shouting but couldn't decipher what they were saying. I was rolled to my side, and someone attached an oxygen mask to my face. Anti-seizure medications were given through my IV as my body thrashed. Everything went dark.

I woke up a couple of hours later to someone calling my name. There were so many monitors. Two tubes in my nose. An IV running in my foot. 'Ahhhhh,' I responded. 'Take it slow,' he said kindly. 'Do you know where you are?' 'Ahhhh,' was all I could say. 'That's okay for now,' he said. No. It was not. I wanted to know what happened. I wanted to tell him I was okay. That I didn't need to be in the ICU. But I couldn't.

The next evening the neurology ICU doctor came in. 'Well, the EEG and head CT came back normal. We're not concerned about any major neurological issues. We think this was just a bad reaction to being taken off your medication. You're ready to go back to the general medical floor.' To me, this was the best news in the world. But my parents looked confused, 'So you don't think there's anything wrong with her? What about...' The doctor cut them off and responded, 'Given the fact that she is now lucid and all her tests are normal, we're not concerned about any major neurological issues.'

I stayed in the hospital for another three nights, and when all seemed okay, I finally got to go home. The doctors had mentioned to my parents the possibility of FND as an explanation for my 'episode'. A psychiatrist and neurologist discussed with them what that meant; however, at that point a reaction to medication change was thought to be the best explanation for my symptoms.

A week later, while eating dinner with my family, I started to feel sick. Everything was spinning and it was hard to catch my breath. I barely managed to communicate that I needed to lie down before it all happened again. I fell into a seemingly comatose state, although I was completely aware of my surroundings. By the time my parents had called 911, I had begun to seize, my body thrashing and barely breathing.

Paramedics arrived and transported me back to the hospital. We were met by an entire trauma team. Once I stopped seizing, they ran more tests, all of which were normal. The neurology team was consulted and instructed the ER team to diagnose me with FND and send me home. We were told that since my symptoms were not life-threatening I shouldn't return to the ER. And that was it. They sent us home, my parents in a state of confusion and fear about my diagnosis. I was terrified. How could my symptoms be psychogenic when they felt so real? I wasn't doing it on purpose or for attention – wasn't that what psychogenic meant? What if the doctors were missing something?

The next morning, I had another seizure. My parents called 911 and I was once again rushed to the ER. My parents insisted on seeing a neurologist, who finally came down to talk to us. She reassured us that all appropriate tests had been done and they were confident in my diagnosis. I was sent home, where I rapidly began to deteriorate.

Before the seizures started, I had been a very active, successful student. I lost all of that in a couple of days. I began to have 15–20 seizures a day, sometimes lasting hours. I developed paralysis for as long as 14 hours at a time, unable to move, speak or swallow. I was taken to four different ERs, over 15 different times.

I began to believe that the seizures were my fault, that I was doing them for attention. It seemed that no one believed they were real or out of my control. No one knew how to treat them. I became suicidal, having lost all that was important to me. I had to be hospitalized in a paediatric psychiatric ward. It was awful. The psychiatric team believed my seizures were for attention and ignored them in spite of the injuries they caused.

My parents searched tirelessly for FND treatment. They probably called a hundred hospitals and clinics, even looking internationally. Finally, they found a psychologist specializing in FND and epilepsy who agreed to treat me. We packed up our car to move to a new city for at least a month.

Even before our first session, the psychologist showed that she cared deeply about me and stopping my seizures. My parents had been told to ignore my seizures by my local hospital, as attention 'made them worse'. However, my new psychologist instantly debunked that theory during our online consultation over Zoom. She taught my parents how to help me return to the present moment and relax my body. The number of seizures I was having declined, improving my quality of life even before meeting her in person. When we finally met, she coached me through recognizing warning signs of my seizures before they happened and using grounding techniques to prevent them from occurring. She helped me examine the root cause of my seizures, and how to cope with my severe anxiety and perfectionism. She helped me unpack my deeply complicated medical trauma from years of living with chronic illness. Most of all, she told me what I needed to hear from the beginning: these symptoms were not my fault, and if I worked at them, I could get better.

From day one she said, 'This doesn't define you. You will get better.' And I did. Within one week of treatment, I went from 20 seizures a day to one a week. After a month of treatment, I went home with much better control of my FND symptoms. The two years since then have had bumps and roadblocks, but I have now been free of seizures for seven months. I can drive, swim in open water, go for runs by myself, and most exciting of all, I am in college. Recovery is possible. Hold on to hope.

2

Facing Mt. Everest

Female, 31 years old, UK

FUNCTIONAL MOVEMENT DISORDER

I have always had a get up and go attitude. Nothing in my life has ever got me down and I never let it. Like most people, I have had my life traumas but nothing that could compare to me having to call an ambulance. I was 20+ weeks pregnant with my second baby, and I couldn't stand up or feel anything from the waist down. It was instant; I didn't realize at the time but I had also peed myself. I was rushed to a hospital with a suspected spinal stroke. This had been confirmed as a minor stroke, but this is where the movement issues of my FND arose. I spent the next ten days learning how to walk. When I was discharged, I could walk using a Zimmer frame [walking aide]. I was totally terrified, wondering what sort of life my children would have. As a massive football fan, my dream was for me and my boys to play football in our garden, and I was faced with not even being able to run after them unaided, never mind kick a ball.

Since then, I have developed arm tremors as well and severe back pain. My sensations are all off as well. When I am standing in the shower and the water is hitting me on my right side it feels as if its burning through the layers in my skin, yet the left side feels as it should. Walking feels as if I'm stepping on glass and nails, but I have learned to grin and get on with it. My speech can also be very poor, yet later in the same day be fantastic. Memory is a big issue as well. I'm grateful I now only need to use a walking stick outside our home. Learning to pace myself and giving up my career has been very difficult. I also feel like a lesser partner, mum, and person as a whole.

I am learning more and more about FND from my neuropsychologist, and finally I have an understanding GP. I still feel as if I'm at the bottom of Mt. Everest looking up, wondering how I will ever achieve this. But my boys give me my strength, they need me. I, like many other FND sufferers, struggle with admitting my issues and why and how I have to pace myself. It can go either way, where people are understanding, or people look at you as if you are faking it all! I just wish it was more accepted, but I am trying to educate as many as I can. If only one person feels less of the stigma I've felt, I would be incredibly happy. The brain truly is the most magical and wondrous thing, but right now I'm so cross with mine.

3

Why I Love Treating FND

Neurologist, eight years' experience
of working with FND, UK

I love being a neurologist and looking after the whole range of neurological conditions that we treat. But most of all, I love treating people with FND. I'm sorry to say that this makes me a bit unusual. Most neurologists find dealing with functional symptoms difficult, challenging or frustrating. When doctors talk about 'heartsink patients', they are often referring to people with functional symptoms. Many neurologists don't even see FND as being their job to treat – even though it's the second commonest reason that patients come to see us.

Why the discrepancy? I don't think I'm especially unusual. Nor do I think that other neurologists are uncaring, unkind or lacking in intellectual curiosity. So, what is going on here? Maybe if we can understand this, we can improve things for patients. Paradoxically, I think that the things I love about FND are actually the same things that many doctors find difficult.

First of all, I love the fact that we can make a confident clinical diagnosis of FND using our skills in history taking and examination. This has always been the essence of the art of clinical neurology. Clinical diagnosis requires a lot more skill than booking an MRI scan or nerve conduction studies. But many neurologists lack confidence in making a clinical diagnosis of FND. This is just because they haven't been taught. I was lucky enough to learn from some of the great clinicians. Now all of us working in FND have a duty to focus on educating the next generation of doctors to make them more confident in diagnosing this condition.

I love treating people with FND because I can really make a difference. There is so much unmet need in this condition. FND is so common and disabling but has had so little attention from the clinical and research community. Most patients experience delayed diagnosis and poor communication from health professionals. Just by explaining the diagnosis clearly, we can make a huge difference to patient experience. It may not seem much – and obviously is not enough for someone to get better – but it can be the first step on someone's journey of recovery. Not knowing how to talk about the diagnosis is one of the reasons that many neurologists find this condition difficult. They're not sure how to navigate the complexity of this genuinely biopsychosocial condition. They're afraid of saying the wrong thing (and often do!). Once again, the answer lies in education. Explaining the diagnosis of FND is not a difficult skill to teach, it's just not usually taught.

But there's more to it than diagnostic explanation. I enjoy getting to know my patients so that I can individualize their treatment plan. I can then support patients to access the rehabilitation approach that is right for them. Many doctors find treating FND difficult because they feel they haven't got anything to offer. It goes without saying that doctors want to help their patients, so we feel satisfied by writing a prescription or performing an operation. It's true that things are not so easy in FND. But actually, we know quite a lot about what helps: a rehabilitation approach tailored to our knowledge of the mechanisms of functional symptoms. The challenge is accessing this in a healthcare landscape where specialist services and expertise are insufficient. Doctors will enjoy treating FND once they can access treatment resources, so we need to be determined and tireless in our advocacy for parity of esteem between FND and other neurological conditions.

I love working in the field of FND because it's such a fascinating condition. Research in FND takes us from advanced imaging of complex brain networks, through novel pharmacotherapeutic approaches to complex aspects of psychology and sociology. Understanding FND may ultimately provide great insights into consciousness and what it is to be human. But for many doctors, not aware of this recent research, FND just seems like a mystery or something that we have 'half-baked' explanations for. It's true that historically we have relied on half-baked explanations. 'Conversion' never really made any sense and certainly didn't explain most of our patients' experience. So, we need more of this great science. As the field advances, there's no doubt that a wider neurological audience will become more interested.

I also love FND because I want to redress the balance for a group of patients who have been neglected and disbelieved. Sadly, many doctors are still influenced by a conceptual model which puts functional symptoms somewhere on a spectrum with feigning. The arguments against this have been eloquently expressed (Edwards, Yogarajah & Stone, 2023) and probably don't need to be made to this audience. But we do need to convince our colleagues. As long as doctors don't fully believe their patients, their patients will not feel believed. And our patients cannot believe what we say unless they feel validated in the clinical encounter with us. The most important message when I teach doctors about FND is just to start by believing your patient.

So, I think all neurologists could enjoy FND and the answer lies mainly in education. It's great to see the trainees I work with doing a better job than the generation before them.

The final reason I love working in FND is our clinical and scientific community. This community is interdisciplinary and has been enhanced and strengthened by working alongside people with lived experience. At the recent FNDS conference in Boston, one of the most inspiring moments was when the audience gave a standing ovation to the amazing @FNDPortal, a person living with FND who shares information, news and their own experiences of living with the condition. With this community working together, I have no doubt that the coming years will see substantial advances in the understanding of FND and its treatment. So, I'm sure that by the end of my career I will love working with FND even more.

Reference

Edwards, M.J., Yogarajah, M. & Stone, J. (2023). Why functional neurological disorder is not feigning or malingering. *National Reviews Neurology 19*(4), 246–256. https://doi.org/10.1038/s41582-022-00765-z

4

Hope and Healing Through Nature

Female, 44 years old, UK

FUNCTIONAL MOVEMENT DISORDER

As I lay in bed, going to sleep, my body softly woke me with small movements, hardly noticeable, and I didn't think anything of it. But they increased and got to the point where they couldn't be ignored. I began to spasm in the daytime, generally while trying to relax, and it became more and more frequent. My physiotherapist was concerned and wrote a letter to my GP.

I set off on a journey of discovery and uncertainty. Google showed me my possible futures, and I did not like what might come to pass. I developed a right-hand tremor and twitched all the time with shoulder shrugs and forward movement in my torso, reacting to loud noises and touch. I rode a rollercoaster towards my diagnosis, and, as a result, my symptoms became more severe. At their worst, they were triggered when walking, hearing loud noises like fireworks, or picking up a piece of paper. I convulsed and threw my arms out in response. I looked like a peculiar air drummer with no rhythm.

The weeks and months dragged past, and I still didn't have a verdict. The stress of never-ending tests, appointments and endless worrying was not good for me. My symptoms got worse.

Work signed me off for a couple of weeks, then more; I eventually took six months off to recover and get my life back on track.

These problems with my nervous system changed my life. For a month, I often didn't leave my flat. I didn't return to work for six months and have never gone back full time. With little information to help me, and in striving for better health, I found ways to keep the symptoms, anxiety and stress at bay.

At every appointment, a different expert bandied about yet another possible prognosis. I hung on to every word. I looked up the terms they mentioned as soon as I could. I grasped at any straw and clung on to any possible hope of finding what was wrong because it might lead to treatment and an end to this nightmare. I wanted an explanation and needed to explain to people what was happening to me. I was told I had epilepsy and then propriospinal myoclonus [a rare condition characterized by muscle spasms]. Both theories were eventually disproven. The whole experience wore me out and I felt as if it would never end. Some days I slept all day, others I wept until the rivers ran dry.

At one point, the consultant invited four colleagues into the room to look at my symptoms because they did not fit their typical list. He asked me to put on a somewhat surreal show. Luckily, like a circus elephant, I performed on cue, and they witnessed the jerky back and arm movements. Their medical discussion passed me by, but the friendly head of the clinic assured me that they could sort me out. So, I just needed to wait for the next round of tests.

Each day, I only committed to getting out for a walk around the docks and river where I'd moved to live with my partner. Even on the days when I couldn't go far, I went to the water to see the horizon and remind myself of the world at large. I set myself the challenge of taking one good photo every day. I became fanatical about small wonders of nature, and they gave me a reason to get dressed and go out. This was no mean feat, as walking triggered my twitches. While I looked and closely observed, all other thoughts disappeared, and the clouds lifted to leave me with a chink of hope. Seeking out these positives played a considerable part in helping me heal. I sensed that, without a break from thinking about being ill and feeling wretched, my body and brain wouldn't be able to move on. It would forget how to be well and get stuck.

Like a bird you can't identify from its distant song, my illness didn't yet have a name and couldn't be seen. My emotions raged like a storm hitting the coast, casting debris and changing the landscape forever. In the end, the clinical tests came to an end and the day of my next appointment arrived.

Again, we entered the neurology clinic with trepidation. With pleasantries out of the way, the consultant informed me, 'It's good news. The tests haven't found anything wrong with you.' Silent tears immediately rained down. If there was nothing wrong with me, how could I be fixed? He seemed taken aback at my frustrated sobbing and assured me that it was a good thing that I didn't have any of the conditions he diagnosed in others. As an afterthought, he sent me to a neuropsychiatrist. The weeks in between the two appointments stretched out and thoughts went through the maze of my mind, meeting dead end after dead end, and never quite reaching the centre. I continued to focus on rebuilding my life, and getting out of the maze, one step at a time.

The neuropsychiatrist told me that I had a functional movement disorder (also known as functional neurological disorder or FND), which was likely to be psychological. I had a diagnosis, but while I now had a name for it, the path back to good health wouldn't be easy.

Had I been diagnosed earlier – before I'd found my own way through – the hospital would apparently have provided occupational therapy, psychiatry and physiotherapy. By the time they told me what was wrong, I was already sorting myself out by other means – counselling, acupuncture and cranio-osteopathy. Happy for me to continue on my own path, they discharged me.

The journey to diagnosis was highly stressful. If I'd been told from the offset what was wrong, then I doubt it would have got so bad. For me, uncertainty bred anxiety and depression, and this in turn made the FND worse.

5

Moving from Despair to Acceptance

Female, 38 years old, UK

MOVEMENT AND COGNITIVE DIFFICULTIES

Fourteen years ago, I fell ill and ended up having what looked like a stroke. I was rushed into hospital, but after a load of tests, lumbar puncture, MRI, CT scan, nothing abnormal was seen, and I was sent home with what they described as a Bell's palsy [temporary facial muscle weakness or paralysis]. But that was just the start.

I began to experience incontinence issues, double incontinence, migraines that would cause stroke-like symptoms, forgetfulness, weakness on my left-hand side, dragging my leg, fatigue, and constant pain but every time I went to see a professional, nothing abnormal showed up in the tests and I started to be told I was manifesting my illness.

On top of my depression, the thought that I was making myself ill pushed me over the edge, and I made an attempt on my life. I was at a really low point. Four years ago, I had what looked like a stroke again, and was sent to the local transient ischemic attack (stroke) clinic. Very quickly, the consultant said that it wasn't a stroke, but she agreed something was wrong, and referred me to a neurologist. I had no idea that the neurologist specialized in FND.

On the day of my appointment, I thought I was going into another appointment where I would be told it was all in my head. That wasn't the case and for the first time in ten years someone listened to me. He told me that he knew exactly what was happening with me and I felt a weight lift from my shoulders. Having a scientific background gave me an advantage in the sense that I understood what I was being told. He gave me research papers and told me it was a marathon not a sprint. I slowly began to understand that it wasn't my fault and that it was okay to have bad days, and to not beat myself up when I did.

I was 23 stone and could barely walk. I used a walking stick, crutches and a wheelchair. My husband had to help dress me and wash me and I couldn't even make a meal. But getting information from my consultant helped me take my life back. I began short walks and after three months of that, the walks got longer. I started losing weight and slowly realized that the exercise was killing the pain. I took up kickboxing and jogging, which some people may think is out there, but it's how I deal with pain. I lost over four stone; I've gone back to work and I can wholeheartedly say that having the support of one consultant helped me understand FND and its effect on me. I have my bad days where I rest up, do nothing, and let my body heal. You never get over an illness like FND, especially when you're constantly in pain. But I have learned to live with it.

6

Sunshine after the Storm

Female, 21 years old, UK

FUNCTIONAL SEIZURES

It all started with a few blackouts and having dizzy spells from time to time, which I put down to stress during the first (Covid-19 pandemic) lockdown. The first GP I spoke to was via a telephone appointment and put my symptoms down to a possible decrease in my blood pressure and said that they would probably disappear on their own. Over the following few months, they got worse, with uncontrolled movements of my limbs and my face, while having what I thought was a general 'pass out'.

After a few months, I managed to get a doctor's appointment and she took bloods, gave me a full health check and decided to refer me to a seizure clinic, which was over the phone. My partner managed to take some videos of my seizure-like episodes, and we sent them over to my doctor. She knew from the first video that it wasn't epilepsy but still sent me for an MRI to be safe. After my MRI came back clear I was then given an appointment for neurology at the hospital, where I was finally diagnosed with FND, or, in my case, functional seizures.

This diagnosis was something of a relief as it gave a name to what I was suffering from. However, it didn't make my symptoms any better or easier to deal with. A few months later, I saw my neurologist for the first time in person. She spent two and a half hours with me (which I wasn't expecting) going over any questions, fears or worries I had and explaining all my symptoms to me in detail. I can't explain the comfort this brought me knowing I had her to turn to if I needed her. I had questions like why did this happen? Can I change anything to help them? Will this get better? Some questions she couldn't answer for sure, but she certainly made it feel less lonely. We spoke about how my mental health had coped with it and how it had affected my everyday life. After the appointment, I have to say that I felt drained. I didn't have a very good few days afterwards. Two days later I had my worst night since having FND. I became quite violent towards myself and had around 20 seizures within four hours. I ended up with amnesia and didn't know who I was, who my partner was or my family. I had bladder retention from my muscles going into spasm, and this lasted for around two hours post seizure.

After that night, I decided to cut my days down at work and focus on getting myself better and having better control of my seizures. The next month, I was hospitalized four times after trying to take my own life. This was my lowest point as I was having around ten seizures a day. I just couldn't control them; I didn't know what my triggers were and I had no warnings to try and prevent them. After coming out of hospital I knew I had to do more than what I was doing, I couldn't let this control my life, and so my dad took me to a therapist. She worked with me to see if I had any past traumas that could have affected me in the present day, which there were.

Having seizures day in and day out put a lot of strain on my relationships, my body, my mental health and my income. My partner and I ended up having a lot of arguments and disagreements, which didn't help the situation. After long months of therapy, neuropsychology, neurology appointments and finding the want to carry on, I'm here today to tell the story. I can't sit here and say it's been easy; it most definitely hasn't been, but with the incredible support of my neurologist, neuropsychologist, my family and my partner, I have managed to have more of a hold on my seizures, and I can now say I don't have ten seizures a day. I have around two dissociative seizures a day and two to three blackout seizures a week. This is a huge step for me. I now work four days a week, I feel as though my relationships have improved and I have a little more independence. I do, however, still struggle with my mental health, but I've come to terms with the fact that life is going to be slightly more complicated with FND and there's always sunshine after the storm.

7

A Psychologist's Perspective on Functional Seizures

Psychologist, eight years' experience of
working with FND, Argentina

During the five years of my career in the School of Psychology, I was presented with clinical histories of people (mostly women) who suffered unexpected attacks, strange behaviours, and exaggerated movements without an apparent cause. These were consistent with Freud's texts that referred to very interesting and flowery clinical cases, sometimes accompanied by images of women reclining on a stretcher with opisthotonos [spasms of the muscles causing arching of the neck, head and back]. When I read them, I was not only transported to the end of the 19th century or the beginning of the 20th century, but also some stories that seemed to be taken from literature, and even science fiction. And that is the way professors explained it to us: that these cases are no longer seen today in clinical psychology.

When I started working in the video-electroencephalography (EEG) unit of a public hospital, I came across patients who had seizures that were similar to epilepsy, but they did not have epilepsy. Neurologists called them 'pseudoseizures'. Then we started to call them 'psychogenic non-epileptic seizures', 'functional seizures' or 'dissociative seizures'. And these patients not only presented with motor manifestations that could not be explained by medical causes, but they also reported complex psychological conditions that reminded me of those 19th-century histories that professors commented on during my degree. 'How is that?' I thought. Today I am surprised that I was surprised. Sure, those stories we read in college were not fiction. They were real. The problem is that by presenting them as a 'historical' condition, almost extinct, there was no need to ask for tools and resources to be able to face these conditions as a mental health professional and help those who suffer from it. With my colleagues at the hospital, we had to start from scratch. We needed to investigate in order to understand. We had to update ourselves on these topics, not only from a theoretical point of view, but also from the technical resources (interventions) of mental health. What do we do? How do we help the patient? Is it helpful to talk? Is psychotherapy useful? Is it enough? Do we need to refer them to another professional? What do they need from us? What should we do and what should we not do? In five years of my career (and many other years of specialization in clinical psychology) no one had prepared me to care for patients with these types of problems or conditions. It was imperative – even ethical – to train ourselves in practices with empirical support that allowed us to help and respond to the patients who came to us.

Even today, many years later, it never ceases to amaze me that, despite the fact that I live in a city with one of the highest proportions of psychologists per inhabitant in the world, it is still very difficult for us to find professionals who are trained to deal with patients with functional dissociative seizures. For this reason, I believe that today the objective is clear: to disseminate and promote the knowledge and training of professionals on FND, train professionals with a critical sense, and promote research into culturally adapted interventions that allow clinicians to respond to the needs of patients. I believe that this last objective is ambitious in the context of a developing country, with few financial resources for research. However, it is a necessary horizon, from the ethical and professional point of view.

8

A Wife's Experience of Stigma

Wife of someone with functional movement,
speech and cognitive disorder diagnosed
seven months ago, Australia

FUNCTIONAL STROKE (MOVEMENT, COGNITIVE AND SPEECH DIFFICULTIES)

When you become a patient diagnosed with FND, it does not really matter what you were before. My wife worked in academia, and I worked in healthcare. That did not matter – our lives, knowledge and experience were disregarded. The stigma was palpable. On one occasion, the doctors on the ward round entered the room, examined my partner, left without speaking to us, and then huddled outside the door whispering. We were told repeatedly that there was nothing structurally wrong. All the tests were clear. When I tried to ask about treatment pathways and allied health input to support recovery, I was dismissed, even though I worked in healthcare and had read the current evidence on how to improve patient outcomes in peer-reviewed journals.

The stigma was multiplied by the fact we were in a same-sex marriage. We lost count of the number of times I was asked who I was. Was I the sister, friend, mother? The confusion when I said 'wife' was clear in the faces of many of the doctors and nurses whose heteronormative assumptions could not fathom a married same-sex couple, plus FND. We do not regard ourselves as 'out there' in terms of lesbian, gay, bisexual, transgender, intersex, queer and questioning plus (LGBTIQ+) politics. However, after my wife had been on a public neurology ward for two weeks, and with us still being regularly questioned about our relationship, our frustration could not be contained. Not only did it feel like we were being regularly dismissed because of the FND diagnosis (and treated as though this was a mental health issue), we were simultaneously othered. Our existence as a married couple seemed to be regarded as shameful and often treated with silence. At times there were apologies, awkward moments when a health professional would realize what they had said and then stutter that they did not mean to make assumptions. But it kept happening. If the treating team could not get this simple detail right, then what other details had not been heard or understood? The ward philosophy of 'patient-centred care' was not the reality we experienced, and we felt badly let down by our exclusion from discussions and decision making.

Some doctors and nurses stood out as beacons of hope, treating us with empathy and understanding – and they were openly critical of the treatment we had received on the ward. At the same time, there was still a general lack of knowledge. If we asked a question, it would often be answered with 'have you seen the website?' (https://neurosymptoms.org or https://fndhope.org). Our answer was 'yes', but these sites did not answer the questions we had, here, now, in this situation. The response in return was often 'well, we don't know much about FND', followed by silence. Our attempts to discuss the current evidence base and options for multidisciplinary rehabilitation and psychological treatment to optimize recovery were met with confusion – it became apparent that almost all staff had very poor knowledge about FND, including how to improve outcomes and effective treatment options.

My wife's sharp intellect and fierce independence had been replaced by neurological deficits, including cognitive confusion, speech difficulties and right-sided weakness. In the early days, she was unable to speak in coherent sentences, hold a spoon or walk unaided. 'I don't understand' became her frequent response to everyday tasks or questions. As time progressed, she (and I) became frustrated, distressed and tearful at her inability to process and understand things which had previously been taken for granted. Spreading jam on a slice of bread and being able to raise her hand to her mouth to feed herself became a Herculean effort; pronouncing words with a 'w' or 'r' seemed impossible until she managed to find her own solution by singing words beginning with those letters and changing the shape of her mouth. We video-recorded key moments when she was able to feed herself and pronounce certain words. These vignettes served as markers on her road to recovery and a means to remind us that there were some improvements.

In the early days on the neurology ward, we were told, 'There is nothing structurally wrong, so you'll make a full recovery and be back at work within six weeks.' In retrospect, this was one of the hardest things to have heard. It bolstered our belief that everything would be okay. We recounted this to ourselves when we were feeling despair... 'Remember, the doctor said you would make a full recovery... It's just taking a bit longer than we thought.' After seven months, my wife is still struggling with cognitive processing, speech and walking, and we now know we were given false hope. Her new treating team are more realistic – she is improving but we do not know the extent of the recovery she will make. The initial false hope means my wife now battles not only with having FND but with an ongoing sense of failure because she was not back at work in six weeks. She still has a long way to go, albeit there have been significant improvements. My wife still cannot leave the house independently, cook, use a computer, write coherent sentences or drive. On a good day, she can walk 200 metres and her gait has improved, but in her own words her walking is still 'not pretty'. She still struggles with stairs, and becomes disoriented and unbalanced by changes in flooring and movement from passers-by. We are not sure when or if she will be able to return to work, and the effect of this long and uncertain journey of recovery and the delay in being offered appropriate multidisciplinary rehabilitation has been punishing on her mental health.

No one wants to hear that they may have a medically unexplained, ill-defined and debilitating illness with a poor prognosis, but even worse than that, one that lacks knowledge and is treated with a lack of care and stigma. We feel let down by local public health services and some healthcare professionals who seemed to put up barriers to care. On discharge, we struggled to get the promised outpatient allied health support, and rehabilitation sessions were stripped back to psychological support only. After declaring ourselves 'desperate' to the neurology consultant, we were finally referred to a private multidisciplinary rehabilitation team. They have provided safe, person-centred care, acknowledging our relationship, challenges and specific needs in a way that makes it feel that recovery might be possible. We have had to pay for this as we were told this level of rehabilitation was not available in the public health service. We do not know what the long-term future looks like yet, but treating people with FND and their carers with understanding, honesty and inclusiveness, and in a timely way, is crucial to optimizing recovery and mental wellbeing.

9

A Nurse's Contribution
to FND Treatment

Nurse, eight years' experience of
working with FND, UK

The role of the nurse in supporting patients with FND is rarely mentioned. However, some of the core skills of a nurse – empathy and compassion, respect, diplomacy, and enhanced communication skills – are all crucial in supporting patients with FND who are frequently stigmatized in very medicalized systems of healthcare. Most patients that I meet who have a new diagnosis of FND have often taken years in getting to that point of diagnosis. They have often experienced a brief and wholly inadequate explanation of their condition and told to go home and read the website (https://neurosymptoms.org). They are also usually discharged at that point and told that there are no specific services to support the condition.

I usually brace myself for a verbal battering during that first contact with a patient. They are often angry, confused and mistrusting of any clinician. I listen to depressingly similar stories of patients being told to 'try harder in physio' (said to the patient with FND who had been a highly motivated long-distance runner until she developed a dense left-sided weakness), or told that they developed the condition due to a brief period of depression at some point in their lives (which is often irrelevant after assessment).

It is no wonder that patients refuse to accept their diagnosis when there is so little education at the point of diagnosis.

I validate their feelings. To be an effective nurse, we need to skilfully engage with patients in a way that develops a therapeutic relationship – particularly within the area of neurological rehabilitation. Key to developing that relationship is understanding the patient in the context of their life history, what motivates them, what their core values are and what they find pleasure in. A healthy dose of curiosity can really develop a trusting relationship.

Undertaking a biopsychosocial assessment is absolutely crucial in being able to understand some of the predisposing factors in the development of FND (in other words, the vulnerabilities). It also highlights the precipitating factors (what was the trigger to the onset of symptoms) and some of the perpetuating factors (what is maintaining the symptoms). For the patient, I have always found that this is possibly the first time that someone has been interested in them as a person, and a clinician is happy to spend two to three hours actively listening rather than undertaking a brief ten-minute intervention. Thus starts the therapeutic relationship of trust.

Discussing how every experience throughout our lives influences the way that our brain develops and functions can foster an understanding of FND and how the mind and brain cannot be separated. I make it clear that FND is an extremely complex condition and one that is extremely individual in terms of presentation, effects on daily life/relationships and in formulating treatment plans. I also like to study their actual medical history as recorded by clinicians and compare this against their perceived medical history. They are often quite different, and this helps in understanding that they may have some strong health beliefs that will need to be unpicked and challenged. There are often numerous other functional illnesses present like fibromyalgia, irritable bowel syndrome, chronic fatigue and chronic pain. There are also often huge amounts of investigations, numerous MRI scans and lots of 'atypical' diagnoses to further fuel certain health beliefs. This demonstrates how medics work in silos within healthcare services and never seem to look at the patient holistically.

I suspect on many occasions, when results from investigations are fed back, it is the medicalized language that is utilized which makes the patient think that an essentially normal scan of the spine (usual normal wear and tear in middle age) equates to spinal compression and severe neuropathic pain. There are also the normal anomalies on brain scans which are incidental and harmless, but when these are discussed with a patient with FND who is trying to understand why they have disabling symptoms, these become their focus and make the acceptance of their FND diagnosis much more challenging.

Trying to demonstrate how the brain frequently goes wrong can be helpful. I discuss being literally 'tongue-tied' with fear or nerves, misinterpreting the weight of an object resulting in using incorrect muscle force (lifting an empty juice carton that you think is full), or being 'paralyzed' with fear. In order to demonstrate the mind/body link, I talk about fainting at the sight of blood, blushing when embarrassed, having a churning stomach when nervous, and feeling sick when watching something disgusting. This can develop a conversation about how the brain constantly interprets information and sometimes misinterprets normal signals as abnormal.

Many nurses in the neurological rehabilitation field have also developed skills and knowledge in grounding techniques, relaxation therapies and educating and advising on strategies regarding fatigue. Stress and anxiety are quite frequent factors in patients with FND, and managing these can help calm the nervous system. Again, education can be key in understanding the two parts of the autonomic system and promoting a better balance between the sympathetic and parasympathetic nervous system. I will often make lots of suggestions, allowing patients to try things and find the tools that work for them. There are lots of mindfulness apps that can teach therapeutic breathing. Things like tai chi, pilates and meditation can be helpful and also offer some distraction. It is important that the patient understands that focusing on movement may result in further weakness, so any distractions, particularly in therapy, can be worth investigating. Discussing possible new hobbies and interests that bring some joy can also be therapeutic, such as gardening, baking or music. Nurses have numerous skills to enhance a multidisciplinary approach to treating patients with FND. Simply listening, developing trust and understanding can be therapeutic/treatment in themselves.

10

Caring for a Loved One with Functional Seizures and Cognitive Problems: A Mother's Story

Mum of a young woman with FND

'Am I dying?' my daughter looks at me, eyes pleading, desperately searching for something, anything recognizable. 'Who are you?' 'Where am I?' she asks, 'What's wrong with me?' The questions come fast and franticly. I hold her hand and tell her I'll explain everything, that she is safe, she is in her own home, and I'm her mum. She is an adult but has the vulnerability of a child right now.

'Am I dying?' 'No, darling,' my voice soft, reassuring, a deliberate hint of a smile in my eyes. I lie beside her, for when the seizure starts this places me in the best position, as I can catch her arm before it starts to pound into her face. I start to explain. 'You have FND, and that stands for functional neurological disorder,' I begin. 'It's a problem with your nervous system and we use the analogy of a computer to explain it. We say it's like your hard drive is working okay but your software is malfunctioning.'

'Why don't I know anything?' I tell her it's a bit like any circuitry, that if a circuit has too much power it will flick the safety switch, and in her case, she has had too much pain running through her system, and it's flicked her memory switch. Analogies seem to work. They give black and white explanations. She wants to know what the terrible pain is, whether she is like this all the time. I tell her she is hypersensitive in every way, to any abnormal or unexpected touch, medication, infection...and that she is in pain, 24 hours a day. Just sometimes the pain is worse, and the memory loss temporarily shuts some of it out. She gives me a look as though I will 'do', mainly in the absence of anyone else and although she doesn't know me, so far, I seem to know what I'm talking about.

'Ooh, my head! Have I had a brain haemorrhage?' I again reassure her, that she hasn't; it's the migraine that comes with the memory loss. She tells me there are miniature men with pickaxes working inside her brain. She feels sick. I reach for the ginger ale, and she has a few sips. Suddenly, the functional seizure begins again. I'm quick and protect her before the blow lands, although her arm jerks out. She's clearly in a huge amount of pain, not in the least because both shoulders have been injured in the past, once by a mugger and the other by a new carer. The seizure eventually stops.

She asks again if she is dying, she feels so terrible. 'It's okay, you can tell me if I am.' She eventually feels sleepy, asks what she should do, and on my reassurance, she gently closes her eyes, passes out for a few minutes, and returns to consciousness. Her memory is back. 'Sorry, Mum,' she always says. The first time that memory loss happened like this, and my own daughter was horrified that a complete stranger was sat next to her (i.e. me), I must confess that afterwards I cried. I took it personally. But as this has happened so many times since, literally hundreds of times, I have managed to desensitize myself to the process and go into auto mode – and that's all it is now, it's a process. Everything that helps my daughter is a process, a way that she, I, or we have developed to help her through a variety of symptoms. Sometimes her memory loss can continue for hours on end; once it was 16 days. Sometimes it's on a loop and the situation above will restart as soon as she comes round again. I am often told that other people don't have the same symptoms as her but, you see, she also has cerebral palsy and two chronic pain conditions. And I visualize the combination of her conditions to be a bubbling witch's cauldron – I can visualize all the symptoms just bubbling up like various potions would, periodically causing some sort of unexpected eruption. Take all her known symptoms and mix them with cerebral palsy, a physical disability that affects movement, and this results in daily seizures and memory loss, always when her body just can't cope with the amount of pain she suffers.

Although many people with FND have comorbidities, I've found little evidence of the study of these when mixed with FND, and vice-versa. So much more is yet to be learned to help people like my daughter. As a carer and a mum, I often look back at earlier times. The days when, despite cerebral palsy, she would go to the gym, we would handcycle miles at night, she would sail, we would enjoy weekends and holidays away. She is pretty much bedbound now, and it's not because of a lack of effort. The hardest thing for her is the loss of what she fought so hard to gain despite her disability. Every day she fights this illness, using pacing and mindfulness techniques. It's not the life she wanted, and it's certainly not the one I wanted for her. I'm only in my fifties, but each day I think about what will happen when I am no longer here, or when I am old. Who would suddenly understand the processes? But, at the end of the day, my daughter is not FND. She has FND, and yes, she suffers from FND. But it does not define her. Every single day I marvel at her optimism, her outlook, her determination to work against this, every single day. Together, we make a great team.

11

Drowning with No Rescue (Art)

Female, 42 years old, UK

FUNCTIONAL MOVEMENT DISORDER

I was diagnosed with functional movement disorder last year.

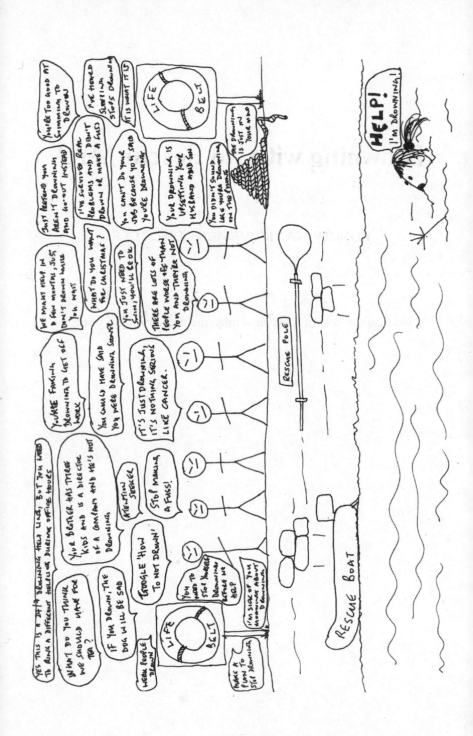

12

Functional Seizures and the Covid Vaccination

Epileptologist and researcher, six years' experience of working with FND, US

As a health professional, I worked during the height of the pandemic, often seeing patients with Covid-19. I worked closely with the hardest hit specialities and witnessed the trauma felt by the other frontline healthcare providers, including internists, emergency providers and nurses. Consequentially, I was one of the first in line for the Covid-19 vaccine and am very supportive of the benefits of vaccination.

As a result, I was anxious when I saw a patient on my schedule who reported new onset of seizures that started within 30 minutes of his Covid-19 vaccination. When reading about the patient beforehand, I saw many features that raised suspicion for functional seizures. My initial fear was that these were functional seizures that started after Covid-19 vaccination and that I would have to talk a lot about misinformation in the media with a patient who was vehemently anti-vaccination. I had personally experienced and heard about many contentious encounters with Covid-19 deniers and anti-vaccination advocates.

When the patient came to my office, I was pleasantly surprised and relieved. The patient was well informed and concerned about his condition. The seizures had a profound impact on his life. He was seeking answers and recommendations for the best tactics to improve his quality of life. When I acknowledged that functional seizures could start after Covid-19 vaccination [not to mean that they could be caused by the Covid-19 vaccine[1]], and that I had heard of that many times before, he was relieved that his experience was both believed and understood. This matched the common relief that I observe in patients who have been told their seizures were fake or voluntary.

In addition, he specifically asked about the risks of the second shot and boosters. Like me, he was concerned about the risk of Covid-19 and wanted vaccination but was worried about it worsening his functional seizures. We had a good discussion about the risks of short-term worsening of the seizures as compared to the risks of Covid-19 with incomplete protection due to only a single vaccination. We made the mutual decision to start cognitive behavioural-informed therapy and specifically prepare coping strategies for when he would get his second shot and boosters. A few months later, I heard that he did indeed get his second shot and there was a worsening of seizures. However, these subsided after a few weeks, and he continued his improvement with therapy. As of today, I have not seen him in more than six months because his seizures have resolved.

Despite my initial fears of a difficult encounter, my experience with this patient who had an increase in functional seizures after the Covid-19 vaccination reiterated the satisfaction that I feel after providing care to patients with FND. The simple act of believing the patient, recognizing the dysfunction caused by their condition, and being able to make a concrete plan to address the seizures goes a long way. In this case and others, there are many success stories of patients improving substantially. This encourages me that my

---

1   Editorial comment – there is no evidence that FND has become more common as a result of the Covid-19 vaccine. For more information please visit: www.neurosymptoms.org/en/faq/covid-19-the-covid-19-vaccine-and-fnd-what-do-we-know.

care and recommendations have a large and positive impact on my patients' lives, which motivates me to continue caring for these patients as well as I can.

13

FND and Chronic Post-Traumatic Stress Disorder

Female, 48 years old, South Africa

FUNCTIONAL MOVEMENT DISORDER

Chronic illness is something I have struggled with for most of my adolescent and adult life. Being sick all the time led me to resign from work after I was only able to work about two weeks a month and I spent the rest of my time recovering. My symptoms varied, including chronic pain, fatigue, and other complications that consumed most of my energy. When I experienced paralysis for the first time, it was from my neck down. Our worst fear was that it may be a stroke, so the ambulance service wasted no time getting me to the closest hospital. In the ER, the doctor ruled out all possibilities including a stroke and infection, and believed it could be an FND. This was confirmed by a neurologist. The nurse assured me that this condition is very real, and for the first time in a long while, I felt understood. I was then referred to a psychiatrist at the same hospital and had to see her the very next day. By the time we left the hospital, my legs were still paralyzed.

My visit with the psychiatrist was helpful. She took a comprehensive medical, psychological and family history of me and how it affected my behavioural patterns. She was knowledgeable on the subject, and as we spoke, I started experiencing speechlessness, tremors and catatonic episodes. These symptoms persisted at home, and it was clear that my FND was affected by my chronic post-traumatic stress disorder (CPTSD), depression and underlying anxiety disorder. Having experienced long-term childhood abuse and neglect significantly affected my mental health and placed significant physical stress on my body. A more meticulous examination to understand my symptoms and create a treatment plan was needed. My psychiatrist referred me to a mental health clinic for a 21-day programme because my symptoms worsened prior to admission. The catatonic states became longer, the tremors and muscle spasms increased and I started having seizures.

At the clinic, I was engaged in various mental health talks and activities, along with creative expression and tension-releasing sessions. My psychiatrist saw me once a day, where she reviewed my progress after psychotherapy, medication and any other required supplements. An EEG was also done, and it came back normal. A psychologist was assigned to help me establish coping mechanisms and prepare me for what I could expect at home, after my discharge. The best method of therapy going forward for me was EMDR, which is especially helpful in treating patients with PTSD. A trauma counsellor who specializes in this therapy was recommended.

From this point onwards, five to six years ago, my symptoms had varying degrees of severity and duration. It was very hard on me, as well as my husband and kids. Finding specialists with experience in FND was also very difficult. Therefore, our GP took over the medication monitoring while my trauma counsellor covered the psychotherapy. For most of my healing journey, I have had to (and still do) draw on my own strength to find the relevant resources in the times I need them most. This can sometimes become a very lonely journey because there is no one to bounce theories off against.

Recovery for me involved addressing my CPTSD, which was like a thick layer of scar tissue formed from all the childhood trauma memories. I had to carefully and gently peel away each layer. This was a difficult and draining process, but it greatly reduced my FND symptoms. Now, I can identify and process most of the triggers associated with the FND episodes. I still experience severe flare-ups occasionally, especially when I'm unsure of the trigger. This has a lot to do with the different layers of fear and how my brain perceives them.

With EMDR, I am able to:

- string all my trauma memory fragments together to form a full cohesive memory
- put the now cohesive memory into the context of my past trauma and allow my mind to process it 'normally' (where it could not before)
- experience the memory as less triggering, and my brain can store it in a 'folder' or delete it altogether
- see the past as the past and the present for what it is now.

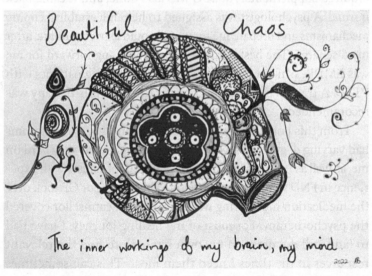

Beautiful chaos, the inner workings of my brain, my mind

Over the last six years, new information on FND and the functioning of the brain-mind dynamic has slowly filtered through on the internet. YouTube became my ally, and when I first heard of the concept of neuroplasticity, a big storm cloud uncloaked from my shoulders! I no longer felt doomed. This gave me the opportunity to search for my own answers and the bright possibility of living and feeling alive again. Authors in this area helped me to listen to my body and to develop a keen knowing of what I need, when I need it. The knowledge about developing new neural pathways drove me to unpack all my board games and puzzles. Little by little, I was able to extend my mental capacities and regain better 'whole-body' functioning (processing language, building connections, movement, sparking creativity, etc.). Coincidently, my husband and I started re-watching our favourite sci-fi shows. In an odd way, the series and characters allowed me to find the language to describe my trauma and experiences to my family. They provided me with new ways of viewing my trauma as I started to identify with the trials and tribulations of certain characters and how they overcame their ordeals and setbacks.

In terms of improving my physical strength through exercise, housework appears to be doing the job for me. It provides enough cardio work, muscle building and strengthening, and mental stamina. It serves as my gauge to monitor my body movements, to see how far I can push them and what my limitations are. My mental stamina and endurance are tested when I complete tasks in manageable chunks, often compartmentalizing them so that I don't push myself beyond my energy boundaries. Striking a good balance and pacing myself are vital aspects.

Where do I find myself today? I am able to manage on my own, with occasional psychotherapy sessions. Although I still zone out sometimes, I am able to bring myself back to my body and the present moment. Performing two tasks at the same time can cause my brain to malfunction, making it difficult for me to understand when someone is talking to me or asking me questions while I am cleaning. Words escape me, and contexts become jumbled, leaving me non-verbal. To fill my days, I engage in creative projects, healing energy practices, and qigong.

Finding FND information on YouTube and the Neurosymptoms FND app has provided me with confirmation of my experiences, feelings and thoughts. These resources have given me validation, compassion, acceptance and a deeper understanding of FND. This has helped my family better understand me during my darkest hours and has made it easier for them to know how to respond to my episodes. Although it can still be confusing for them to understand why I say 'I'm okay' when I have severe muscle spasms or a pain score of 10, they are learning when to respond casually and when to take me to the hospital.

The most important message I have learned is to pace myself on the good days, try to do some activity on bad days, and get enough rest to avoid a major crash. I hope that sharing my story can help others in their journey with FND. Thank you for your support.

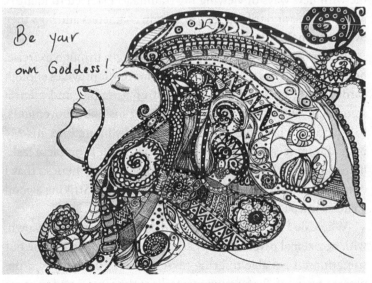

Be your own goddess

Be your own goddess

Sections of this chapter have previously been published in the journal of the South African Depression and Anxiety Group, *Mental Health Matters*.

14

Getting My Life Back

Female, 55 years old, US

FUNCTIONAL MOVEMENT DISORDER

This is my story.

When I was in my twenties, I was diagnosed with myoclonic epilepsy. Myoclonic means sudden muscle movement. This diagnosis was made at a university hospital. My symptoms started with my head jerking as I fell asleep at night. The movements increased to my head jerking during the day and my right hand flailing. For the first five years or so, I tried a variety of anticonvulsive medications. The cocktail increased as well as the side effects, but I continued to have breakthroughs. Eventually, I decided to go without medicine. And mostly it was manageable. Stress increased my symptoms, but then they would let up. That was up until recently.

My symptoms increased to the point that I thought I might have to quit my job. I was having thousands of movements a day. I also added some new ones, such as a bowing kind of motion that made walking difficult, and my head nodding up and down. I wasn't getting much help from my doctors where I lived, so that's when I decided to go to a specialist service in another city. The first week I was there they undiagnosed the epilepsy. I had not had an MRI in 25 years, and the new scan immediately showed that it was not epilepsy.

Then they scheduled another week of appointments and

decided that it was a functional tremor or movement. I actually cried with this diagnosis. Not because I didn't have epilepsy, but because I felt as if I should've been able to control it if it was functional. I felt as if I'd caused it. As if it was a weakness within me. My specialist neurologist suggested a programme consisting of a type of therapy. They said that it could take up to a year to get into the programme. Thankfully, there was a cancellation so I could receive it earlier. The programme mainly consisted of occupational therapy and physiotherapy appointments. I learned guided meditation and nerve glides [which help to restore mobility to the nerve], which helped the most. By the end of the week, I was 85–90 per cent better.

It's been over five years since I was at the programme, and I am still doing very well. I may go several weeks, even up to two or three months, without a functional movement. I think of myself as 'in remission'. The great thing is that I have my life back.

15

A Teen's Experience of Functional Seizures

FUNCTIONAL SEIZURES

Author's mum

This is my daughter's story of living with FND for over three years. She is now 15 years old and wanted to submit her account as she feels it is difficult to find information written by teens about FND. She has seizures most days at school and missed out on two years of her education due to this. She is improving with psychological treatment and support at school.

Female, 15 years old, UK

I developed FND when I was 11 years old. Fresh out of primary school, I had one 'normal' month of secondary school before being launched into a world of functional symptoms. What started out as innocent fainting spells evolved into violent seizures, migraines and episodes of paralysis. After several visits to A&E, I eventually got diagnosed with FND. I count myself as lucky because I received the diagnosis only a month after my first seizure, whereas many others have to wait several months or even years!

I'd never heard of FND and was convinced I had epilepsy.

It didn't help that the doctor in A&E didn't explain it in a good way. My 12-year-old self heard the words 'pseudoseizures' and immediately thought that the doctor thought I was putting it on. He explained that I was 'just' anxious and that I was essentially okay. I just needed to be referred to the Child and Adolescent Mental Health Service. If only it was that simple! In my experience, when professionals use the term 'pseudoseizures' they generally don't have a good understanding of FND. I even had a psychiatrist tell me that 'pseudoseizures' weren't real! Due to the unbearably long waiting list at mental health services, my parents took me to see a lovely private psychologist. Sadly, the support he was able to give me was not enough and my seizures did not improve.

At this point, I was being sent home from school every day due to the seizures – my life was pretty much only FND. I lost all sense of who I once was. I wasn't a sporty, cheerful girl anymore. I was the girl with FND. No one at secondary school got a chance to see the other side of me, only the FND me. At 13 years old, I fell into severe depression. I wasn't a person anymore. I was just a body with FND. Everything was bad. I felt that there was no escape. A few months later I found myself sitting on the wrong side of a wall on a bridge. I felt that FND had won. I didn't have enough support. I'd run out of courage. Life was not worth living if I had FND. I ended up in a psychiatric ward with my depressive episode. I won't go into detail about the whole stay, but my FND was at its all-time worst. I was having over 30 seizures a day, with one day having over 50! This was no life for a 13-year-old – suffering from severe FND and missing out on education.

After being discharged, I slowly started to recover. This was two years, part of which was during the first [Covid-19 pandemic] lockdown and honestly, that lockdown came at the perfect time. I was too unwell to get out of bed but as we were in a pandemic, there was no need to get out of bed. No one did any schoolwork (the world was too crazy, and school seemed like such a minor thing to everyone), so all the anxiety about school was gone! My local mental health service team had started seeing me and I reluctantly began taking anti-depressants. The effects were almost unbelievable! I could think! It was like getting glasses. Everything is fuzzy without them, but when you put them on, everything is crystal clear. As my mental health improved, so did my FND. I haven't had a paralysis episode in over a year, and I've only had one migraine since I've been on medication.

I was referred to a specialist consultant psychiatrist who treats children and young people with FND. Medication combined with amazing support from him have really helped my symptoms. I managed to get an education, health and care plan (EHCP) to help me at school and I now have a learning support assistant with me to assist if I have a seizure. Before I had the support of an assistant, teachers used to stop the whole lesson to help me, but this is no longer needed. Having an EHCP has allowed me to remain in a mainstream school despite still having frequent seizures.

A trigger for my seizures and other FND symptoms is noise. I've never liked noise and I find it difficult to cope in noisy, crowded places, like school corridors or classrooms. I now wear ear defenders in these situations, and they help me to cope. Another way I prevent seizures is by using sensory items. Anything spiky or textured is extremely helpful. Ice packs are great for getting me out of seizures! We worked out that the strong scent of eucalyptus oil works well as a grounding technique. It is still difficult for me to prevent a seizure but as the years have gone by, I've become better at it. I frequently struggle with fatigue and joint pain. Weighted blankets help with both, and I wish I had discovered them sooner! I try to have periods of down time to help with my fatigue. I can do more in the long run if I take small breaks throughout the day. It is no use pushing myself too hard and then feeling as if there is a cloud in my head for the next three days!

I have found that managing FND is a balancing act. One of the things I wish I had known when I developed FND was to not let it become the focus of my life. I became much happier when I stopped letting it control me and did things that I enjoy. As I said before, I lost all sense of who I was. I am now working out who I am and who I want to be and I feel grateful that I am fortunate enough to have been given the tools to do it. I'm no longer only a girl who has seizures. I'm a horse-obsessed girl who loves watching *The Office*, who may also have the occasional seizure. FND is a part of me, but it is not the only part of me.

16

The Unexpected Gifts of FND

Female, 56 years old, UK

FUNCTIONAL MOVEMENT DISORDER

I am a woman with a condition called FND. A stranger to me at first but now we are very well acquainted! A little bit too much I would say. Let me tell you where it all began.

At 49, I was a very fit, healthy woman, loved the gym, had a good job and still had quite a few ambitions left to fulfil when, after a routine operation, my whole world changed. Left with a tremor and odd sensations, I didn't feel like me, nothing was right. No one knew what was the matter with me. I had become quite the celebrity in my local hospital; health professionals came to see me from different specialities, 'Oh you're the lady who had the stroke' or, 'We heard you'd had a lack of oxygen to your brain.' I lay there feeling like I was a medical oddity. The lady in bay four with the strange symptoms but nothing showing up on any tests, of which there were many! What was happening to me? What were they going to do with me? Well, they discharged me, that's what they did. I was sent home in a wheelchair to get on with my new life, with no help at all!

Eventually, bit by bit, I got my strength back. I could walk but was wobbly. I went back to work. 'Yes!' I was getting my old life back! But oh no, 'Bam!' things were getting worse. I couldn't do my job properly, I couldn't function. Access to Work were great and really helped but then it came, the dreaded suggestion, 'I think you need to call it a day now, you've done as much as you can.' Ill-health retirement came to call.

No job, no career, and feeling useless. By this time, everything seemed to be affected: my ears, eyes, brain function, walking, shaking and the dreaded seizures, oh the seizures! It was a seizure that took me to A&E; this same seizure took my legs away that day, the day before my 50th birthday. 'Happy Birthday' FND said, 'Here you go!' From that day to this I've never walked, never felt the floor move under my feet, never stood up to hug my husband again, never been able to even move my legs to get rid of the cramps that hurt so much! Then, here you go, have another massive seizure. This time it took my speech – took it for six months. I was lucky, as my neurologist sent me to a rehabilitation programme for four weeks, but I had a choice to make. What was more important to me, walking or talking? They would only have time to concentrate on one. What would you choose?

Well for me, definitely the latter. Surprising, isn't it? It surprised me too, but not being able to talk, wow it's a killer, believe me. Not being able to express myself with speech made me feel as if I was a nobody. Well-meaning people talked for me at first, then slowly, gradually they didn't talk for me but talked over me, until I was a shadow of my former self with no personality of any recognition, not even to myself anymore. *But*, miracle of miracles, the wonderful speech therapists got me talking again but WITH A FOREIGN ACCENT?! What the hell? Funny and tragic at the same time!

So here I was, talking funny and not being able to walk, partially sighted, two hearing aids, tremors, brain going AWOL and a lot of other weird stuff that kept appearing every so often. The last thing FND gave to me is total incontinence, which is now controlled by a catheter stuck in my tummy! The joys of FND! The gift that keeps on giving. But for all the things FND has taken away from me, believe me when I say it's given me far more. I was forced to slow down. It gave me patience, gratitude, a stillness in my life, the ability to see things in a different way and an appreciation of me, just me, being who I am. Acceptance of a new me, a different me but still a very worthy me with new ambitions. Welcome to my new life. So come on FND, bring it on, I'M READY!

17

My Sister's Brave Journey

Sister of someone living with
functional seizures, Argentina

FUNCTIONAL SEIZURES

The experience that summons me to write these words dates back to over eight years ago, when my 17-year-old 'little sister' suddenly began to have these rare episodes where she lost consciousness and passed out for a certain amount of time. I remember the initial bewilderment, not understanding what was happening or what those episodes were that were so out of the ordinary. Then there was the anguish that this generated for us as a family, for me as a sister and especially for her.

At the speed of light, these episodes began to happen repetitively, occurring up to three or four times a day. I remember at that time hearing sudden noises in the house, some object that had fallen to the ground along with her or simply her body falling on the floor in a new faint. Sometime later, I noticed how my mind had associated those unexpected noises with the outbreak of a new episode, making me react to go to my sister when perhaps it was just a falling plate. The repetition of those very distressing episodes made my brain associate those sounds with seizures.

In the course of two or three months, our lives had gone from ordinary to crisis ridden. My sister went through a diagnosis of epilepsy that, fortunately, very quickly was ruled out to affirm that her episodes were 'psychological'. At that time, we did not understand anything about it. She would pass out, move her body in strange ways, shake, her eyes would roll back, she would bite her tongue and contort. At times, she simply remained silent, as if 'asleep', or would hum a song and say words and unconnected phrases that could last for an hour. I still feel in my body the anguish and despair of not understanding what was happening, not knowing how to solve it or how to help, not knowing what the future was going to be like, and realizing that she could find herself without warning in a situation of such vulnerability and exposure.

At that time, we did not have much more of an explanation for the episodes than the fact that they were psychological, as if her mind dissociated in the face of emotions that overwhelmed her. The years passed, the series of episodes fluctuated, there were different medical studies and different professionals – until last year. New seizures appeared and, after investigating, my sister found specialized professionals who made the diagnosis of 'non-epileptic psychogenic seizures' within the spectrum of FNDs. Throughout this process, I saw my sister battle between anguish and the desire to get through it. There were moments when bewilderment and uncertainty crushed her spirits. Depression and anxiety appeared, and along with each new seizure was the anguish of not knowing what her life was going to be like, if she was going to be able to build the life she wanted, if she was going to make her dreams and desires come true, what her condition meant. And in the midst of that rough sea that she sometimes still sails (and we sail as a family), her strength and her courage appeared as an anchor that we have learned to take hold of and trust.

Every time I see her small, vulnerable or despondent, she surprises me with her resilience, her courage, her ability to face the difficulties that the diagnosis presents her with, but which are far from being impediments. I see her so whole, having grown so much with each setback. I don't know if this experience had anything to do with it or not, but she has developed such a clear sense of what she wants for her life, along with the tools that have allowed her to start building it. This experience has been, and may continue to be, a huge challenge for all of us as a family, for me as a sister, but mainly for her as a protagonist. It is one of those experiences that leaves you raw, feeling with every millimetre of your skin everything that your condition as a human who experiences suffering implies. And it is precisely for this reason that I believe that travelling this path has awakened in each of us a more human, more sensitive, side. Being vulnerable, afraid or suffering is what makes it possible for us to be brave and act with courage – fundamental attributes for building a meaningful life. And that is why for me, the bravest person and the one I admire the most in the world is her, my little sister.

18

Brain Overload

Female, 54 years old, US

FUNCTIONAL MOVEMENT DISORDER

Why will this dizziness not go away? Why is it so hard to walk? So many questions... This is how my story begins.

Several years prior to the start of my symptoms, I went through a very emotional traumatic situation not knowing that is where it all began. My symptoms began several years later, out of the blue. When my symptoms started, I went to my doctor, who ordered a variety of tests, which all came back normal. I was referred to another specialist who ran more tests and, again, nothing was found. I was then sent to another specialist for more testing. I've had countless investigations. After a period, I was again sent to another specialist, who thought it could be either seizures or migraines without aura, and I was started on a medication. Within two days of beginning the medication, I began having non-stop shaking in my arm. The next day, my whole left side was shaking, my arm would fly up above my head and I had no control. With each step, my leg would go much higher than it should before it would come down to take a 'step'. Then it moved from just my left side to everywhere, all extremities, and my head just bobbed non-stop.

I went to the doctor and was told my body was adjusting to the medication and to keep taking it, and it was important that

I did not stop it. After a full week of this, I started feeling as if I was losing my mind, I couldn't keep my train of thought, nothing was making sense and I told my husband to take me to the ER. There, they told me I was having a severe reaction to the medication, and I needed to stop taking it immediately and never take it again. Because my heart rate was so high, I was advised to see a cardiologist. When I saw the cardiologist a few days later, I was still having movements and I was told to go home and pack a bag as he was admitting me to the hospital.

Once in the hospital, I was told I had sudden onset of Parkinson's disease, which was later ruled out. I was then told it could be Huntington's disease and they'd need to contact an outside lab to confirm, which could take up to three weeks. Also, after yet another brain scan, they thought I wasn't getting enough blood to my brain so they did an angiogram. During that test, they confirmed the blood flow to my brain was working properly. After a few more days in the hospital and more tests, I was discharged with a diagnosis of conversion disorder.

I was to follow up with my local doctor and when I did, conversion disorder was something they had not heard of. I immediately got to see a psychologist to assist me with everything going on, as this was all very stressful.

Because I would not accept this diagnosis, over the next few years, I spent a lot of time seeking second opinions. I struggle with motor dysfunction, balance and dizziness the most. Out of nowhere, I lose control of my left arm or leg, and I can't stop it. Or sometimes my head will not stop bobbing up and down. I just have to laugh (or cry) and call myself bobble head. It's just part of the disorder and there's nothing I can do until it passes.

My symptoms can strike when I'm anxious, or when I feel no anxiety at all, and that part is so frustrating. Just being in a different surrounding can set it off: a loud sound, music, lighting are all triggers for me. My therapist calls it brain overload. When a trigger sets things off, things go downhill very quickly. I absolutely love music but over the years I can barely listen to it and when I do, it must be very low which is very different from my younger days!

I seldom go anywhere because through the years of this, I developed severe social anxiety and panic attacks, something I never had previously. Even if I'm excited to get out and go somewhere with my husband, usually within five minutes I get overwhelmed, and the symptoms take over. I can look forward to something for weeks and when it gets to the day, the FND tells my body 'Nope, not today'. I get dizzy, my legs can't seem to remember how to walk, my arm or leg want to start flip flopping like a fish, my head bobbles nonstop and I get facial tics – the list can go on and on...

I have named all my movements with silly names like bobble head, loosy goosy for my neck, flip flops for my arms and legs, but hey, I have to keep it positive as this can really bring me down at times. The disorder impacts me physically and mentally. My movements and mobility can fluctuate from minute to minute; therefore, I no longer drive. I have had physical therapy to try and help with my balance disorder; however, when it flares up and until it settles down, there's not much I can do except to practise my exercises, practise positive affirmations, and wait it out, which takes anywhere from a few hours to a few days. It's never the same. During the days following an onset of symptoms, which I call my recovery days, I am just flat out exhausted. I need almost complete silence, or very quiet surroundings while my mind and nervous system get back in sync.

It took me several years to accept this diagnosis, but each doctor I went to for another opinion confirmed it.

We never knew this disorder would change our lives so drastically. All my hopes for things I wanted to do at this time in my life... Well, I can sit and wallow in my self-pity for days. It can be a very isolating disorder. I cannot go into a restaurant, a mall or a movie theatre, as all are huge triggers for me; however, I do try occasionally, even though often it turns out to be a failure, with lots of tears, sometimes downright sobbing, but I don't give up. It affects not just me but also my family. For many people with FND, their family and friends cannot understand or accept this disorder and that can be very isolating. I am thankful for my family, who have helped me when an episode starts as sometimes it's very difficult to put words together to talk, and they know what to do, without needing to ask anything. For me, it's very hard to socialize; and making plans involving time is extremely difficult. But I'm fighting and I refuse to give up.

19

I Feel Like I'm Drowning; Trapped in Myself (Art)

Female, 39 years old, US

FUNCTIONAL SEIZURES

I was diagnosed with FND 12 years ago.

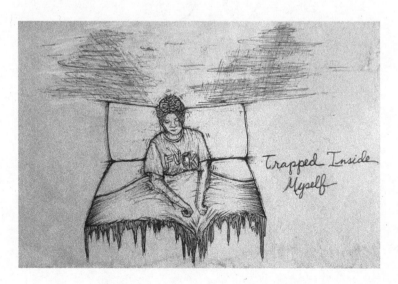

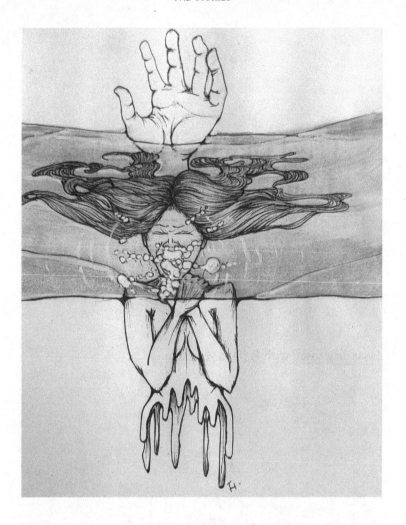

20

Learning to Adapt

Female, 42 years old, UK

FUNCTIONAL MOVEMENT DISORDER, FUNCTIONAL SENSORY DIFFICULTIES, FUNCTIONAL COGNITIVE DIFFICULTIES

How did I go from an independent, confident woman to being unemployed and struggling with daily life? FND! Never heard of it? Neither had I. Two years ago, I was doing a charity walk. I had only completed about four miles when my left eyelid felt heavy. I carried on walking but then had to stop. I had pain through my body, my left side felt weaker. I thought I'd had a stroke. This is really where my FND journey began.

I was rushed to hospital and had MRI and CT scans. I couldn't stand properly and my speech was slurred. I was terrified as it was during the Covid-19 pandemic, and I couldn't have anyone with me. After two days of examinations from the neurologist, I had my diagnosis. I really had no idea of the impact it would have on my life. I was allowed home after four days but there was no support given. I was directed to a website and just left to it.

Everything was so unknown. How long would I be like this? My speech was worse, I couldn't get words out and when I did, I was stuttering or getting them wrong, so communicating was a nightmare and exhausting. I was scared to leave the house as I'd lose my balance and fall. The continual dizziness when standing

81

was sickening. Pain in my legs caused me sleepless nights but my nightmare was just beginning. I couldn't get to my work and therefore I had no income. Having to rely on family and friends for financial support was embarrassing, given the fact I had worked since I was 12. I was no longer living but existing. I was at an all-time low. I became isolated and had never felt so alone. I just didn't know how I was going to carry on like this. Nobody could give me answers. It was always you may or may not improve. I seemed to spend days crying, grieving for the life I once had. I'd enjoy going to work, the theatre and singing. I was out more than I was in, and now felt trapped. I struggled to eat meals as I could no longer chop vegetables or stir something in a pan due to tremors in my hands and pain being elevated. I was having panic attacks out of nowhere, and then I had to call an ambulance for the first time as I thought I was having a heart attack.

I had to do something, so I self-referred for counselling to enable me to cope. These sessions were difficult as it relied on me being honest about previous things I perhaps hadn't dealt with in full. I always had this 'just get on with it' attitude but never really dealt with how events had made me feel. Now I was forced to re-live it all over again. What it did make me realize was that I had come through the other side of those dark times, and I could again. So what could I do? I'd lost my job as I was unable to get there and could no longer manage the work so all I had was time. With no community health support, I started my own daily routine of therapy. Small exercises to move my legs and arms. Singing out notes and sounding out vowel sounds to improve speech. Playing scales on the piano to improve coordination, and although it was tiring, I persevered.

My speech has got better. My attitude towards my diagnosis has changed. I'm embracing this new version of me. Yes, I experience difficulties day to day but I'm learning to adapt so I can overcome hurdles. When I'm in pain, I've found that art is a great distraction technique, and relaxing. I struggle to concentrate as I get blurry vision at times, but meditation helps alleviate this symptom. I can suddenly go deaf depending on noise levels, but my hearing eventually returns. I still lose my balance, but I try to focus on one main spot to steady myself. On particularly bad days, I have a walking stick with me for support, so I feel more secure. The tremors come and go. I have not found a solution for stopping them, but relaxation does ease them more quickly. I've adapted the food I buy, such as buying pre-chopped items, and I use a slow cooker, so I don't have to worry about stirring. My memory is an issue as I struggle to remember things on a short-term basis. I've found I need notes and to set alarms on my phone as prompts, which does help. I know I have a long way to go but I'm determined to start living again.

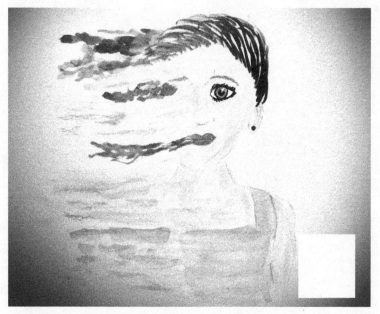

Art by the chapter author

The worst thing about FND is that nobody sees it. You are made to feel like a fraud, from strangers on the street, family and friends to the gruelling benefits [welfare] system. You are already fighting to just make it through each day without breaking down in tears because you don't want to live like this, so having to justify yourself to other people is exhausting and degrading. The best method I've found is to concentrate on the things I can achieve rather than the things I find difficult, therefore I never feel like a failure. Support groups online are helpful, but I have to be wary of becoming bogged down with the negativity or struggles other people face, which can affect my mood too. Living with FND is an uphill battle and unless clear pathways across all hospital services are equal, with no postcode lottery, there will always be people like me who feel let down. We can all be warriors with the correct care and vital support.

21

The Winding Road: A Wife's Story of Functional Seizures

Wife of someone with FND, UK

FUNCTIONAL SEIZURES

My husband was diagnosed with FND four years ago, after quite a lengthy process over a number of years of going back and forth to various medical specialists. It's fair to say that he was getting quite fed up with the 'it's not this' and 'it's not that'. From appointments with consultants, blood tests, cardiac tests, then moving on to inpatient EEGs, then on to ambulatory EEGs and finally, finally getting a diagnosis and being able to put a name to 'it'. While it might have seemed like a relief to start with, FND is really not a 'one size fits all' finding.

Prior to his diagnosis, he had been having a number of regular functional seizures, or 'wibbles' as we named them, over a number of years and they still continue. They vary from a disassociation that can last a matter of seconds, a 'back in the room' moment; or longer term, to more major attacks that can simply floor him for days. I've become adept at seeing the signs: how his speech is affected, how he can stagger. It's as if he is drunk, but without the alcohol. He can get the functional seizures at any stage of the day and has also been known to get them when he's asleep. It's been all-consuming though, as he is no longer able to work. Our dog too can recognize that all is not well and will stick to his side like glue when an attack is imminent. The simple act of petting the dog is soothing and helps de-stress him. Pacing daily is an art form, and perhaps it's not one that he's perfected fully yet.

He is learning to live with FND and I suppose he doesn't really have an option. It's part of him now and he tries not to let it control him, but it does affect what we can and can't do. He doesn't like crowds and lots of people, as it makes him anxious and stressed, which in turn can bring on an attack. Familiarity is good and reassuring, so we end up going to the same places on holiday, rather than going somewhere new. Perhaps his avoidance of social gatherings is now a learned behaviour. We used to love going to music concerts and rugby games, and while we can still do these activities, we have to be a bit more considered about them.

From my own perspective, FND is part of his make-up and part of the man that I love and have known for over 20 years. Yes, it's a pain, and yes it can cause mood swings and anxiety and yes, it affects what we do, and how we do it, but we've learned to adapt and work round things. I don't suppose we've really got a choice in that. Nothing is unsurmountable, even if the road might be a bit more twisty and windier than we'd anticipated.

22

A Quick Guide to the FND Journey

Male, 56 years old, Australia

FACE TWITCHES PLUS COGNITIVE DIFFICULTIES

Part 1

My symptoms are face twitching, stuttering and cognitive difficulties. Stopping work and eliminating stress from my life were the keys to managing my FND. No more face twitches, though I still have cognitive difficulties. I'm not sure you ever get 100 per cent better, but you can manage your FND and move on with your life.

My contribution is a short list of points that I wish someone had given me two years ago when I developed FND, kind of like a very, very quick guide to the FND journey. Here's what I've learned:

- FND is a strange little thing, and it takes a long, long time to understand and accept. You can't rush getting better.
- Talk, talk, talk. My neuropsychologist is fantastic at this, as is my neurologist. And, speaking of them...
- You need a team! Professionals, family, friends. It might take you a few goes to find the right professionals, but keep at it.

- Only you know you. Meaning – take as long as you like and say no whenever you need to.
- Pace yourself, but always have improvement as the eventual goal.
- Know your triggers. I wish I knew this on day one! I think this clicked with me about a year or so into the whole process.
- Once you've identified your triggers, address them or remove them. I know that sounds incredibly simple, and it's not going to be feasible for everyone, but it was the one giant step for me on the path to improvement. If you met me on the street now, I don't think you'd even know I had FND. I'm not better though, just different. And that's just fine. You learn to accept it, manage it, and move on the best you can. Here's how I describe my FND to people now: essentially, there's an imaginary line of what my brain can and can't do. If I stay on the good side, then I'm fine. If I get close to the line, I'll start to stutter, cry and get confused. I don't work anymore (that is simply beyond me), and I don't drive anymore (my brain could get overloaded and freeze), but life is still good.

If you're on the journey, there is light at the end. It's a tough, shitty, exhausting journey, but you can get there. Good luck!

Part 2 (ten months later)

I'm sitting down to read this for the first time since I wrote it. It's so interesting to look back then and compare it today. Then, I thought I'd peaked on my 'get well' journey. Now, I've made significant life changes that have helped me enormously.

So, an update! First, I've started driving again, which has improved my life immensely. Second (as suggested by my neuropsychologist), I've started boxing. I don't have the reflexes of a 20-year-old anymore (who would at 56!), but it's a fantastic (and fulfilling) physical and mental workout. I box twice a week and love it. And lastly, I've started exercising more (other than boxing) and am feeling on top of the world.

I'm also seeing a counsellor every two to three weeks (for, as I call it, a 'mental health check-in'). I now know my brain and body better than ever, and if I can get plenty of rest and sleep and avoid my triggers (super-busy environments, stress!), then life is good – easily the best it's been since this all started three years ago. I'm finally feeling like my old self and am getting better every month. I'm sure there'll be a few unexpected hurdles again (as FND seems to do), but until then, onwards!

23

My Wobbly Brain

Female, 44 years old, UK

FUNCTIONAL MOVEMENT DISORDER

I am married and have the most amazing little boy who is disabled. I am also living with FND and have done so for the last three and a half years. I have struggled with very little understanding or help from most healthcare professionals. It took me a lot of courage to ask for help and when I did, all I got was closed doors.

It all started with a pain in my face. My son was due a medical treatment and when I spoke to the GP about my pain, he said it was the stress of that, which at the time made sense. The pain didn't go away, in fact it got worse and no matter what the GP gave me, nothing helped. My son had his treatment, and he was in casts on both legs, which meant me lifting him in and out of his wheelchair. I was in a lot of pain.

Three weeks after his treatment, I woke with the most intense pain in my head. My husband drove me to our nearest hospital many miles away and by the time we reached it, I had lost all feeling down my right side. We live in an isolated area so it's a small hospital. It was decided that I needed to be taken to a bigger hospital. I went the following day and got lots of tests straightaway.

After a week, I was diagnosed with FND after the Hoover test [test used to identify functional weakness]. The neurologist came to speak to me and asked for my phone. I handed it to him.

He typed in a website and handed me back my phone and walked away. I was left to get home by myself with no help from the hospital. I feel I have been left like that since my diagnosis. Every time something goes wrong, I get told, 'Oh, it's due to the FND'. I feel as if I have been left to get on with my life by myself with zero support.

I can honestly say, FND is the worst thing and the best thing that has ever happened to me: worst because it's totally changed my life, but best as I've met some amazing warriors along my journey. My fight is far from over, but I feel I have learned how to deal with my new life, and I will even use the word 'disabled' to describe myself, which I feel is a massive step for me. Since I have accepted my diagnosis, I have started using photography to help me through the hard times and this has now led me to raise money from selling my photos and it is going well. My son and husband have accepted my 'wobbly brain' and deal with it the same way I do, day by day.

24

Left Without a Pathway

Female, 36 years old, UK

FUNCTIONAL SENSORY DIFFICULTIES

My symptoms started with joint pain and initially I was referred to rheumatology. I had investigations with no known cause. I then woke up one morning to find the right side of my face felt numb. We were in the middle of the Covid-19 pandemic and I was so worried I was having a stroke. I rang the GP who got me to check my facial muscles in the mirror and he wasn't concerned. My head also felt all fuzzy. The following morning, I woke with the same symptoms but now my right leg was numb too. My husband took me to A&E where they took some bloods and said all tests were clear, but they would refer me for an MRI scan as they wondered if I had multiple sclerosis.

A few days following this, I ended up bedbound. I couldn't eat. I was really dizzy with the fizzing feeling in my head and was so fatigued – like never before. I spoke to the GP, who sent me to an out-of-hours GP as I felt so poorly but I got told it was probably viral. This episode lasted six weeks. I then returned to feeling normal, but my symptoms came back six months later. It was the same as before: bedbound, stroke symptoms, fuzzy head and fatigued.

My GP then made a referral to neurology. I was so worried I had multiple sclerosis. I started googling symptoms and treatments preparing myself in case this is what I had. My MRI appointment came before my neurology appointment, so I had a scan of my brain. This was useful as the results were ready in time for seeing the neurologist. He told me it was clear! I was convinced he must be wrong as I had felt so ill. How could it be clear? He then did a physical examination. He mentioned that he thought it was something called FND. I had never heard of it. He wrote down a website and sent me home. He said he would see me again in six months.

I had mixed feelings. I finally had a reason for all my symptoms, but I was in denial, and I was convinced they were missing something. What if I had a brain tumour? I battled through the next few months and returned to see my neurologist, telling him my symptoms were persistent. He said he would repeat the brain scan but also scan my spine and use contrast which gives a clearer picture. I felt happy that things were getting double checked. Again, the scan came back clear.

Now was the time to accept my diagnosis and take some action. I joined an online support group and realized there were so many others like me! But also, so many people worse than me. This scared me as I then had the worry that I may get worse. I asked the neurologist what I could do to help relieve my symptoms and he suggested psychological therapy, which was an online course to help deal with health conditions. I followed his advice and although it was interesting, things didn't change for me. He told me he would refer me for another type of psychological therapy, but this had a two-year waiting list, so I paid privately and had some other types of psychological therapy. This has helped me deal with the condition better, but my symptoms continue.

The hardest thing about this condition is that there is no pathway. No treatment plan at all. You have to fight for help and treatment. The GPs are not educated on FND and, like most people, have never even heard of it. How can they support us if they don't know anything about it? I'm lucky in the fact that my GP has listened to me on my bad days and has offered medications to help some of my symptoms, but I mourn my old life and the hardest thing is that each day is so unpredictable and there is very little support available. The only support is friends, family and the online peer group, which is a charity run by volunteers who have FND themselves. Surely there should be a service available where there are healthcare professionals to contact, as there is if we had multiple sclerosis.

So that's my story. I live with FND every day. Some days are better than others, and I have to cherish those days, but the bad days are really hard and lonely. I'm grateful for friends and family as without them I don't know what I would do, but unfortunately some people don't understand. You find out who really cares and I'm truly grateful for those who do. I'm also grateful for my neurologist, who listened to me and did the appropriate tests to get me a diagnosis.

25

FND Shame

Female, UK

FUNCTIONAL COGNITIVE DIFFICULTIES

Functional Neurological Disorder Shame

Kids, gym, fun, and the odd migraine.
But a change of medication decides to mess up my brain.

Face looks like a stroke but need to rule out MS [multiple sclerosis].
Go private for a brain scan, but no damage...adds to my stress.

You're just depressed, go on meds they'll sort you out.
Here's a website, go see for yourself what FND is about.

That's not treatment, I've a list of symptoms three pages long.
I have children, help me, did I do something wrong?

We only help people with neurological symptoms we know how to treat.
See a shrink, left to feel I'm crazy, pain, tears, just incomplete.

How can I not remember my own children's names?
No money coming in and somehow trauma is to blame.

I was happy, I had a life...please someone help me.
I had confidence, could remember, even have a degree.

95

Broken, nothing working. Who calls this functional?
Exhausted, no job, healthcare so untouchable.

Three years on I write in desperation to a neuro in my local area.
Listened to my symptoms, seen me as a person not just hysteria.

It didn't matter to him the reason I was in his chair.
He listened as I sobbed, finally...someone cared.

Read books, YouTube, Facebook in my search for info.
Need benefits, pace myself, where did the old me go?

Friends deplete, you look normal, there can't be much wrong.
Exhausted, in pain, stay in bed all day long.

A different life, lift myself out of the trashcan.
None of this was in my bucket list or my lifelong plan.

Medical apartheid, post code lottery for treatment, fights along the way.
An end to stigma, isolation, shame...hope this happens some day.

26

A Black Hole

Female, 31 years old, UK

FUNCTIONAL MOVEMENT DISORDER

It took five years to get a diagnosis and following that, my whole world changed. FND felt like a black hole had been swallowing me for five years and I didn't even know what it was. It became a spectre living on my shoulder every day. When you get your first symptom, you dismiss it as you 'slept funny' or you are feeling a little run down, and then over time, you realize it is more than that and something just isn't right.

I was terrified when I got my diagnosis, I thought I was losing my mind. Test after test came back normal and I started to question my own sanity. Having FND has so many limits but over the last few years, developing coping mechanisms and identifying triggers have made a scary illness slightly more manageable. It never goes away but celebrating the small wins, like only having one episode of weakness today or not losing my speech, may seem like a small victory but for me it is huge. I don't want anyone to feel sorry for me, I am a warrior every day. I am an FND warrior.

27

Coping with FND

Female, 59 years old, UK

FUNCTIONAL MOVEMENT DISORDER AND FUNCTIONAL SEIZURES

This story is my FND journey so far.

Four years ago, after a usual week of being at work, while sitting watching television, my right leg suddenly had a life of its own. Trembling and shaking, it was as if the leg momentarily didn't belong to me. I laughed it off. However, a few days later it happened again and so began the doctors' appointments to discover why, at my age, this was suddenly happening.

During the following couple of months, and being unable to work, my symptoms increased to seizures and dystonia. I was prescribed medication to help relax me and a muscle relaxant, which 'knocked me out'! I continued to have blood tests, GP appointments and then, after an MRI, an EEG and a day in hospital, I was diagnosed with functional seizures and FND. I was told to read all about it on https://neurosymptoms.org, the medication (which I hadn't been on for long) was stopped and I was informed that I would be referred for neuropsychiatry and put on a waiting list.

Going out of the house on my own was impossible and I missed being able to walk unaccompanied. I now had a wheelchair and avoided seeing people. An outing was a trip to the GP for regular

98

vitamin injections, which were subsequently stopped when my level went too high. Having a very understanding and compassionate manager, it was agreed that I would return to work in a minimal way on days I felt I could manage. At that time, this was a huge step yet seemed a little ridiculous that, having previously held a senior role at work for 30 years, I was potentially about to return for a few hours and only 'if I could cope'. This did give me a focus, although some days proved too much and recovery between was spent in bed with fatigue.

Six months later and with unpredictable symptoms of seizures, gait issues and arm weakness, I got a call to say I could start neuropsychiatry sessions and CBT. Sadly, after completing the six-week course, I did not experience any improvements and was back on the waiting list for a follow-up appointment and review. During the following months, I developed a hoarse voice and stammer along with my already existing issues. I felt as if it was a spin of a roulette wheel each day as to which symptoms I would suffer. Trying to maintain a positive attitude and a sense of humour was getting harder, and I didn't often consider the impact it had on my entire family. I felt at a loss as to how to help myself and kept clinging to the fact that I was going to be seen by a neuropsychiatrist again. This time, having done my research, I wanted permission to get an appointment with the specialist team at a specialist hospital. My prayers were answered when, at my review, it was agreed that I should be put forward to go to this hospital but with an understanding that the waiting list was very long.

A little over three years after my first symptoms, and following an initial assessment at the specialist hospital, I finally received a call for a five-day course of neuro-physiotherapy to start. This proved to be very beneficial, and although I still require a wheelchair and my symptoms remain, it helped me with coping and management techniques, leaving me feeling more hopeful for a brighter future. My treatment is ongoing and my FND journey continues. No reason has been found for its onset. BUT, I feel incredibly lucky to have been diagnosed and to receive help in what, for this condition, is a relatively short time…and I still manage to work for a couple of hours a week.

28

Sensory Strategies

Female, 48 years old, Australia

FUNCTIONAL MOVEMENT DISORDER

I live with FND and also observe patterns of others' FND in online groups we are in together. I'm not a trained expert, but these are just things I've observed.

It seems clear to me, in layperson's speech, that FND is a disorder of brain overload. When someone with FND experiences brain overload in a way they are particularly vulnerable to, their neurological symptoms intensify and diversify. The ways someone can be vulnerable to brain overload tend to remain fairly constant for each individual, sometimes increasing over time. Brain overload leading to neurological symptoms can be caused by things including temperature (heat, cold, fever), physical tiredness, mental tiredness, pain, stress, hormones, being asked too many questions in a row, trying to communicate about a difficult topic, repetitive movement, trauma, past trauma being triggered, sensory sensitivities and sensory processing disorders (sound, light, smell, taste, feeling on skin), an attack on the immune system, comorbid conditions flaring up (like depression, diabetes, or obsessive compulsive disorder), sudden surprises and so on.

It is extremely beneficial for each individual with FND to pinpoint which things cause their particular brain overload, and work to limit those in their life. This may help prevent FND from increasing and diversifying in symptoms exponentially, or at least it can help to reduce symptom flares. I do think it's most beneficial to people with an episodic tendency in their FND presentation to do this, but I'm convinced it can lead to significant neurological symptom reduction for most people with FND.

At my worst, I was bedridden for three years and eight months with paralysis and severe limb weakness (sometimes I could only blink and breathe), acute sensory processing disorders, swallowing and choking difficulties, speech difficulties, incontinence problems, an eating disorder, migraines lasting up to 30 days each, three different injuries in one shoulder from my condition, and I had a time of severe stress on top of severe stress and I had two violent and extremely painful functional seizures as well.

It has also been incredibly beneficial for me to engage with sensory activities which do soothe and bring me joy: ceramics or easier polymer clay or air drying clay; drawing; colouring; collage; playing with my hands in water, even in the sink; raised garden beds I can access in my wheelchair so I can plant and pick flowers and vegetables, and sit and watch the pollinators attracted to the flowers; photographing flowers and architecture on walks in the wheelchair with carers when I'm able to get out, or photographing flowers in my garden; patting my cat; playing the piano softly; putting fingernail stickers on my nails; peeling or cutting an orange, or having it peeled or cut into sections for me and smelling or eating it; carrying a small sensory box with me at all times, full of tiny items to choose from to soothe my senses when I'm feeling overloaded, like scratch 'n' sniff stickers, mini scented highlighters, smooth milk glass to look at the world through, wishing pebbles to hold, velvet ribbon to run through my fingers, essential oil roll-on, popping candy to taste, sticks of good tasting gum, miniature books to look at, quotes I love, a beaded woven ring to wear and so on.

When I was bedridden and my limbs were almost completely paralysed except my hands, I had support workers put a tub of art supplies on my lap, and a pair of scissors and glue, so I could make tiny, collaged books. I sent the books to friends who needed encouragement. Creating a bubble of peace around me which I can control and from which I can connect with people (mostly online) has been essential to me in taking step after step to build up strength again to get out of bed after living in bed for so long. I tried physiotherapy, and any repeated movements I concentrated on immediately increased my paralysis and severe limb weakness long term. I've done CBT in the past and it had no effect on me at all. Mindfulness made me anxious unless it was activity based, as in sensory activities I could be present in. I have an extensive trauma history, but taking a step away from that and focusing on peaceful living and joy in my life now, what I can create, how I can support others with art, and gardening, has helped more than anything in settling my trauma.

Knowing I have the ability to replace one thought with another gives me a lot of control over my past. I choose to write it down or tell it to my psychologist if my trauma flares up, then to refocus back onto soothing activities and connection with the now and others. I was hospitalized repeatedly for depression in my life, but my depression has completely stabilized and actually gone with this focus on sensory activities and peaceful living which I now have. I have hope because I know I have the power to take a step right now to separate from something which overloads my brain, towards something which soothes my brain. I know it isn't a big wondrous miracle, but it's one tiny step after one tiny step in the right direction, with as many rests as I need in between. Not beating myself up. Just a gentle, gradual journey where I look back regularly to notice the changes.

I wish I could share this with everyone who is struggling to know what to do for their FND, alongside any other medical and allied health support they are receiving.

29

Managing School with Functional Seizures

Female, 20 years old, UK

FUNCTIONAL SEIZURES

I was 16 when I fell ill on a residential trip and ended up in hospital for a week. I was throwing up violently and having these episodes where I would violently shake uncontrollably. I had various tests, but there was nothing unusual. The doctor put it down to an infection from the lake we had been canoeing in during the trip. I was discharged.

Less than two months went by, and I had my first seizures – I have no memory of what happened during them at all, and they began with no warning at all. It was scary because I was in my first year of sixth form and having anything from seven fits a week to six fits per day. The school could not handle it and told me that I'd have to do my work from home as they couldn't deal with having to call the ambulance every other day and it was disturbing other students. That really hurt. It evidently resulted in me having to drop a subject as there was only so much I could do to teach myself at home. All the while, I had these constant tests and trips to A&E until one doctor decided that it was probably just epilepsy and gave me medication for that. The medication did not work and caused more problems, from extreme tiredness to excessive swelling of my limbs and the deterioration of my mental wellbeing.

I was eventually taken off the medication as there was no clear evidence of epilepsy and it was doing me no good. After various hospital stays, an EEG and an MRI, I was seen by a neurologist. She had no idea what was happening and because I was a teenage girl, she put it all down to stress. After a few appointments, she stopped seeing me. During this time, I was also referred to an eye specialist as my eyes were not coordinating with each other – another MRI was done to rule out internal damage. Then I had a test done with a fine wire that went across my eyes to test how well they worked. They found some slight damage to the optic nerve, and I was then given some advice on how to improve this and continued having regular appointments.

As I hit the age of 18 and all these appointments continued, my friends at school were confused as two years had passed and I hadn't been diagnosed with anything, but I was still having these episodes and going to the hospital for various appointments. A year passed and nothing; I was beginning to think all was well but then I had another seizure. I was disappointed that what I'd thought was gone, was just lying dormant for a while. I turned 19 and eventually got another neurologist appointment and was finally given a diagnosis of FND but that was it. I wasn't told anything about it. What it was. If there was anything that would stop it. I was left to research that myself. All the while this was happening, my eye appointments continued, and no significant change happened. I am now waiting for surgery to hopefully resolve the issue. My functional seizures still occur, though not as often as before. New symptoms and diagnoses I have received are migraines, dizziness for no apparent reason and random chest pains with no explanation.

I am now 20 and at university, trying my best to not let this disorder define me. My goal in life is to prove that even with a condition that is complex and sometimes frustrating, I can achieve everything a completely normal individual can. I hope that in the future there may come a day where someone can tell me exactly what I can do to put a stop to this condition but for now, I'm just trying to live my best life.

30

A Poem: I Have FND

Female, 59 years old, UK

FND, INCLUDING SENSORY DIFFICULTIES

Functional Neurological Disorder Poem

'Are you ok?'
'Urm, yes I'm fine.'
'You don't sound it.'
'Yes, I'm fine.'

Why didn't I tell them I'm not fine?
Why do I not say 'I'm not fine?
I have FND.'

'Are you ok?'
'Urm, no I'm not.'
'Oh, what's wrong?'
'I have FND.'

'Oh, you look ok.
You seem ok.
I've not heard of that.
What's FND?'

'When did you get it?
How long 'til you're well?'
'Its cause isn't always known,
No treatment either.'

'How are you today?'
'Still not well.'
'You look ok.'
'I have FND.'

'I can walk well some days and others not.'
'Oh, you seem ok.'
'Oh, but I'm not,
I have FND.'

'I can't stop today.
Got things to do and people to see.'

'I wish I could do things today,
Not rest and pace.
I struggle some days,
I have FND.'

'I haven't been out for days,
I'm tired and ache.
I'm lonely and bored.
I have FND.'

'I'm fine' I say.
'Oh, glad you're better.
You look good today.'

'I'm glad I look good,
I'm sad, I don't feel it.
I am tired and frustrated,
I have FND.

I miss my old self,
Who was capable and well.
I miss my old life,
I miss the old me.

I have lost some friends,
And gained some new.
On my good days I'm fine,
You'll see me outside.

I've had to leave work,
But do other things.
On my bad days you won't see me,
I have FND.

So when you see me, don't assume
That if I am out, I am better, because I'm not.
I just live with my FND.

I have good days and bad.
I struggle a lot.
Just because you've not heard of it,
I still have FND.

I live with it.
I hate having it.
I have to accept it,
I have FND.'

31

The Challenges of Functional Seizures

A psychologist, two years' experience
of working with FND, and neurologist,
20 years' experience, Brazil

FUNCTIONAL SEIZURES

'Are you a psychologist? Then, please follow me quickly,' the nurse urged. It was seven years ago, when I was working in a public hospital in Brazil, the largest country in Latin America. As soon as I arrived at the ER, I was startled by what I saw: a middle-aged woman, shaking intensely from head to toe. Her hands and feet were twisted as if there was an invisible force pulling them towards her body. Her chin was shaking so much she could barely speak. They were trying to sit her in a wheelchair. I didn't know what it was, but one thing was certain: the patient was terrified and so was her family. The nurse in charge came up to me and whispered in my ear, 'It's a case for you. It is a conversion seizure.'

She was my first patient with FND (at least that was the diagnosis she received). The only knowledge I had on the subject came from a distant undergraduate lecture, when the professor warned us: 'Be careful! Many cases are misdiagnosed as conversion disorder', and then she told us the story of a patient later diagnosed with a brain tumour. That was it. The one and only piece of information I had, in fact, was a counter-example. So, I took a deep breath and, armed with my single tools – welcoming and listening – I went to meet the patient. I tried to do the best I could.

Luckily for the patients, I would have the opportunity to improve my skills shortly after, when I started my doctorate studies under the guidance of a team of epileptologists in an epilepsy comprehensive care centre in Brazil. The challenge was enormous. I didn't know anything about it. My supervisor and her teammates didn't even call this condition the same thing I had learned about. They used the term 'psychogenic non-epileptic seizures' (PNES), also known as functional seizures. At first, what were just two different names later became 199 distinct ones. Yes, our research group has catalogued exactly 199 variations of the name in the English language.

Nowadays, after consulting my former colleagues from university days, I realize that I wasn't the only one who was out of the loop. I found that most of them had never seen or at least recognized a person with FND. In the rare exceptions, they had seen at most solely one case/patient. Therefore, some questions popped up in my mind: 'Why have almost none of my fellow psychologists seen people with FND? Has this disorder practically "died" along with Freud? After all, how many people are diagnosed with FND? Where do they go for help? How do professionals make the diagnosis? How do they treat it? Why did that nurse deprive the patient of hearing the diagnosis when she whispered in my ear? How did the nurse make the diagnosis? Did the patient receive the correct diagnosis?'

Under the guidance of my thesis supervisor, I am slowly discovering the answers to all these questions. The answers are not always clear or easy. They are not always satisfactory. For these cases, we reserved a privileged place in my thesis and persevere in the search for better answers. Even with two years to go before completing my studies, I have no doubt today that my first patient with FND would find me now much more prepared to care for her.

32

Childhood Trauma and Stress

Female, 50 years old, UK

FUNCTIONAL MOVEMENT DISORDER
WITH VOCAL DISTURBANCE

I always thought I had good mental health. I had survived ten years of sexual abuse as a child by three different relatives. As an adult, I had 'dealt with' the issue by reporting the perpetrators to the police and seeing them receive prison sentences. In my late twenties, I lost my baby who was stillborn, and I was unable to have any more children. I had ongoing physical health issues thereafter, but I prided myself on how well I had coped with my life's experiences.

I've always been a very active person. I completed a mountain-eering challenge for fun and try to walk at least 10,000 steps a day. I used to swim regularly and could swim a mile with relative ease. I've always enjoyed working and have had a variety of jobs. It was while I was working as a manager in a fairly high-pressured role that I first noticed some changes. I snorted a lot, mainly when I laughed but it became a daily occurrence. I also often had painful joints and used various support aids.

My grandmother died while I was working there, and, looking back, I recognize that my FND symptoms started around that time. I felt vibrations running down my legs; I kept checking my phone thinking I had received a message, but there was never any-thing there. I've always been clumsy, so tripping up and banging into things was normal for me. I lost my voice periodically, putting it down to laryngitis [inflammation of the voice box]. It usually happened whenever I had a cold or infection, so I never thought much if it.

Unfortunately, I was made redundant and had to find a new job. I found a job I loved, working with people with physical disabilities. I worked there for almost ten years. The manager bullied most of the staff. I think he saw a vulnerability in me and as his threats and demands increased, my stress levels went through the roof. I started stuttering, my left hand and foot went numb, and I had continually painful joints. I used a stick to walk and couldn't enjoy my daily walks. My GP referred me for investigations for multiple sclerosis, which came back negative.

Two years ago, I had a flood at home, was facing redundancy again, Covid-19 rates were rising rapidly, and I got a chest infection. I woke up and my voice had gone. Nothing unusual. I tried to get out of bed and couldn't. My partner had to half carry me to the bathroom. Initially, I thought it was a side effect of the antibiotics I was taking at the time, but after two weeks my symptoms were getting worse. I felt as if I had spiders crawling on my legs and arms. My ankles, knees, hips and hands were so painful I had to use a special pillow between my knees at night. I had migraines that made me vomit and I couldn't think clearly. It felt as if someone had given me a strong sedative. I've always slept a lot, but I couldn't keep my eyes open! My sentences were muddled – my family knew what I was trying to say so it wasn't too much of an issue.

After struggling like this for two weeks I spoke to my GP. Covid-19 meant they were avoiding seeing patients face to face, but my doctor asked me to come in. My symptoms were mirroring a serious health condition Guillain-Barré [a rare condition that affects the nerves], so my GP had me admitted to hospital. After seven days of every test you can imagine, a neurological physiotherapist sat with me and asked if I had experienced a childhood trauma. I explained that I had, but that I didn't understand why he was asking. He said that he and a multidisciplinary team would have a chat to discuss their findings.

My consultant, physiotherapist and speech and language therapist explained that through exclusion of other conditions, I had been diagnosed with FND. Up until that point, I had no experience of FND. It didn't make sense. Why would my brain create such problems for me? It seemed like self-sabotage. While lying in bed, I was able to move my legs but not when I stood up. That showed my legs were working, which I think helped me get my head around the diagnosis.

My physiotherapist got me a frame and helped me shuffle a few steps. We tried to climb a few stairs, but it was impossible at first. Covid-19 rates were rising rapidly, so we mutually agreed I would be discharged and would have physiotherapy at home. This didn't happen because of the Covid-19 infection control restrictions, but I did the exercise programme daily and went for walks at midnight, so people didn't see me shuffling along.

I was discharged to my partner's house, which is on one level and had a shower rather than just a bath. He had to help me with all aspects of daily life: personal care, dressing, cooking, shopping – I couldn't do anything without assistance. This frustrated and distressed me and I cried every day.

I developed a vocal tic, a whooping noise which happened hundreds of times a day for around five months. I was scared that the tic would stop me doing things I enjoy – I go to a lot of lectures but would have been too embarrassed to attend. People stared at me on the bus and in shops. I shied away from talking to people who know me.

Luckily, I was able to work from home because of the Covid-19 lockdown and was considered 'vulnerable' and advised to shield. This meant I was able to 'return to work' remotely. I tried to carry on as normally as I could. I explained to people about my tic and people were very understanding. Once shielding finished, I returned to my workplace. I used a four-wheeled frame to get there and back. Sometimes I couldn't walk at all, so I got my partner and friend/colleague to help me get on and off buses in a wheelchair.

I spoke to my GP, who prescribed a medication commonly used for depression and we found a dose that helped. It also stopped my migraines! My partner was amazingly supportive and researched ways to help. He understood that my symptoms were rooted in my subconscious, so asked me to imagine that my brain is like a clock – if you open the door, you can see the workings; when you close the door, the clock still works but the workings aren't visible. I visualized sweeping out my brain and locking the door behind me. Honestly, the tics stopped that day! To work on my mobility, we tried dancing, walking with my eyes closed, anything to reach and interact with my subconscious mind.

My partner said that he had read that a type of psychological therapy can be used to address PTSD, so I asked my GP to enquire further for me. I was assessed by the mental health team at my local hospital, and it was agreed that I would be a suitable candidate for it. I had ten sessions which were intense and hard work, and my symptoms greatly improved!

I learned to keep my stress levels down with breathing exercises and I do a Sudoku before I go to bed – this takes the focus away from any worries I might have before I sleep. I make sure I get enough sleep and use the FND app that my consultant recommended. I attended an online FND seminar, which was very informative. Little things like having heavy shopping delivered have also reduced my stress levels. My partner, family and friends have been amazingly supportive, and I am grateful that I have them with me on this journey.

I found a new job, which I absolutely love. While I have some ongoing FND symptoms, they are manageable, and I have been able to get on with my life. I recently had a dinner party and went to an art exhibition. I no longer use a stick and can easily climb stairs.

I finally feel like 'me' again – the key for me was understanding the condition, recognizing the triggers for my symptoms, and reducing my stress levels by doing things I enjoy. I work with my brain now, rather than fighting against it, and am at peace with my FND.

I hope that sharing my experience has helped you in some way, if you think ' that sounds like me!', to show that there is hope, that you can live a 'normal' life with a job, and a social life and do the things that make you feel happy and fulfilled.

33

Trying to Cope Without Support

Female, 55 years old, UK

FUNCTIONAL SEIZURES

I was diagnosed four weeks ago. This is my story.

At the start of the year, I started to notice that my left arm was behaving weirdly. It was making moves independently and not stopping. A few weeks later, I experienced my first 'seizure'. I went to the local hospital where the doctor listened to me talk about my symptoms, did a quick examination, and then said I needed to be seen by colleagues at the seizure clinic and to call my own GP to ask them to do the referral. I was told 'no driving and no work' until we had a better idea of what was happening, but to go straight to A&E if I had any more seizures.

On the following morning, I contacted my GP to explain the situation and ask for the referral to be sent to the clinic. The doctor I was talking to said she would not refer me until I had been seen by her. When I asked why, I was told that this was the practice. So having seen the doctor at the hospital, I was now slightly confused as to what my own doctor would find that he hadn't. On reflection, I called the GP practice again and asked to speak to another doctor. While waiting for the call back, I had another seizure so off I went to A&E again.

While being triaged, my own GP practice called to apologize for the confusion, the doctor had been wrong, and they had made an appointment at the clinic for me. The team in A&E were great, they did blood tests, a full history, a CT scan and a CT scan with contrast – which showed no tumours or signs of a stroke. They advised me to rest at home until the appointment at the seizure clinic and if I had any further seizures to come straight back. The next day was great as I had no seizures, I was just tired. Then came the next day, when my husband found me on the kitchen floor seizing, with one of our dogs watching guard over me. My husband called an ambulance and by the time they arrived the seizure, which had lasted for about 40 minutes, was coming to an end. So off to A&E again, this time in an ambulance.

After my initial intake, they asked for a neurologist to come and assess me. The doctor did a neurological exam on me and told me that he thought I had FND. I had never heard of this; however, when we went through my recent medical history, permanent left-sided headache, weirdness with my left eye – it feels like it is blind, even though I know logically that it isn't – left-sided weakness, falls and bumps for no apparent reason, exhaustion after doing most activities and spending most Friday afternoons and Saturdays sleeping because I had been in work earlier in the week (for my job I spend a lot of time on my feet), plus other symptoms that I had just put down to being stressed and tired, his diagnosis did seem to fit. The doctor explained that what I was experiencing was real and that it was the software part of my brain not working properly. He gave a website address for https://neurosymptoms.org and said he would arrange a follow-up appointment with another doctor in due course. With that I was free to go home, and this is when I began to struggle with the whole concept of FND.

I am a type 1 diabetic and from diagnosis onwards there has been support, help and advice available whenever it might be needed. I see my team at least once every six months and have regular blood tests to make sure everything is okay. My insulin control is tight, mainly because I need to reapply for my driving licence every three years, and I have been determined to keep it. With FND though, there was nothing except a website, and being told I needed to inform the Driver and Vehicle Licensing Agency as I would not be able to drive until I was three months seizure free. There was no one I could call to ask if the feeling that my left leg was being dragged behind me was normal, or to talk to about the balance issues I was having (I look as if I'm drunk when out walking), or my right eye starting to feel weird, or the overwhelming exhaustion that comes after a seizure, or the fact my arms feel they have no power in them. The best they could give me was an appointment at some point in the future; they couldn't give me an idea of the date as they were so busy. This feeling of helplessness had me questioning the diagnosis, trying to stop myself from having the seizures (which in my experience didn't help) and not resting when I was tired, as this was a sign of weakness, in my opinion.

So, what have I done? I have joined a number of support groups on Facebook, gradually begun to realize that I have no control over this disorder (hard to do as I am so obsessive and compulsive about my diabetes) and found, completely at random, two other people who have this disorder.

What lies ahead? I have no idea; I am determined not to allow this condition to define who I am. I have my youngest son's wedding this year, as well as a trip booked with my oldest son and his wife. I know there will be days that are more difficult, but I am ever hopeful that these will become easier to handle as I continue to work on accepting FND.

34

Balancing on the Tightrope

Female, 36 years old, UK

FUNCTIONAL MOVEMENT DISORDER

Functional neurological disorder. Three words that on their own are comprehensible, easy to understand. But together, the words form a medical diagnosis, one that has become an enigma and is often misunderstood. Its symptoms are usually invisible, hidden away but can suddenly appear as if conjured by a magician, becoming visible and making their presence known to everyone. Living with FND, I feel I am constantly walking a tightrope, balancing between the kingdom of the well and the kingdom of the sick. If I stumble one way, my illness remains secret, an invisible secret only I know. But if I teeter the other way, the symptoms I try to hide become visible, revealing my life with FND. It is both a blessing and a curse when the symptoms of FND remain invisible, known only to me. It's a blessing that the illness, symptoms and resulting limitations do not define me and are not the first thing people notice. It allows me to choose who to confide in about my life with FND, and when and how.

I find that people do not hold lower expectations of me or are not limited by popular stereotypes or sweeping generalizations when symptoms are invisible. It is a blessing that others often don't notice; makeup can help hide the dark circles under the eyes and conceal the other visible effects of living with a debilitating illness. I like that I can paint a smile on my face to trick those who don't know me well or the struggles I endure because of living with FND. It affords me 'normalcy', being able to weave in and out of the realm of the able-bodied as I please. It allows me to act and fake being well. But it is just that – an act. I regularly pull off a performance to make everyone believe everything is fine. But in truth, every day is a fight, a constant battle, trying to keep that smile fixed on my face. But often, the demands of FND and its accompanying symptoms supersede everything else, and this performance becomes difficult to sustain. And the struggles that I try so hard to hide are suddenly exposed.

One of the most frustrating curses of living with FND is its tendency to be invisible, concealed from the outside world. Then, it is easy for others to dismiss my symptoms or downplay their existence as being 'inside my head'. It is frustrating when everyone assumes that I am coping without seeing how heavy the demands are every day. A constant source of frustration is the inability of others to witness the fight I endure every day; the failure of others to see all of the ways FND affects every facet of my life. These invisible battles and the lack of understanding from others only add to the loneliness permeating my already microscopic world. You don't see that I am faking being well, faking being healthy to preserve my dignity, energy and ability to accomplish whatever I have planned before my legs fail me and I collapse to the ground. But you don't know the effort it takes to fake being well. And although this performance is challenging, it is often easier than exposing the pain that exists and having to use precious and already limited energy to defend my permanent state of being unwell. What you don't see are the grimaces I make behind closed doors, a safe place where I feel comfortable removing the mask I wear in public, and I can allow myself to acknowledge the unrelenting, debilitating pain. The pain I constantly attempt to conceal when among you, the healthy. You don't see the overwhelming fear and anxiety that creeps into every aspect of my life.

The fear is that the list of existing limitations will continue to get longer, and the number of losses will increase exponentially;

the concern that I will continue to worsen. And the worry that FND will eventually become the sole existence of my life, and I will end up all alone in the world because of it. You don't see the anxiety and fear that begin to stir up when having to leave the house. The fear that symptoms will suddenly appear. You cannot know the self-doubts that continually creep in; doubts of what I am capable of and over-analysing and questioning every decision. I often overestimate the extent of my limitations, regularly convincing myself that I cannot do something or handle going somewhere because of the disabling symptoms that exist because of FND.

You don't see the excruciating pain that greets me in the morning. Or the number of times it takes for me to even get out of bed. You don't see as the weakness in my legs prevails and they refuse to work. You don't observe the nights my body contorts from unrelenting pain that radiates down my spine and throughout my legs. You don't see me as I cry in bed, the days and nights with my arm in my mouth, trying not to scream from the all-consuming pain. Or the days spent crying or feeling anger at everything I can no longer do and everything I have lost. You don't see the constant dizziness and vertigo that consume my entire life. You do not witness the unimaginable struggle of walking or standing in a queue when my legs shake, trembling, so relentless that it is the only thing my mind can focus on. You do not see the unimaginable anxiety that courses through my mind that my legs will suddenly give way, leaving me collapsed in a heap on the floor. You don't see the incredible loneliness that I feel because of FND. The friends I have lost along my journey of trying to fit into a world where I seemingly do not belong. There is a lot you don't see about my life with FND. But for me, it is for real and highly debilitating.

35

Managing Energy with Functional Movement Disorder

Female, 63 years old, US

FUNCTIONAL MOVEMENT DISORDER

The sun was shining through my window when I awoke. I was grateful to wake up rested and refreshed and looked forward to spending the day outside. Winter is slow to depart where I live and today promised to bring a breath of spring.

Anticipating spring's arrival and impatient for it to begin, I had already bought a collection of fruit trees and berry plants to begin a garden and orchard on the property where we had just moved. They were waiting in the garage for a day nice enough to begin planting. After breakfast, I headed to the garage to start work. I looked over the group of trees and berry plants and was surprised to see how much I had bought. It would be easy to wear myself out if I wasn't careful. Since I have FND, I have to use my energy wisely so I don't compromise my function.

I was thankful to be having a good day. Some days it wouldn't be possible to tackle such a daunting task. The day before, I had mostly rested. We had thrown a 96th birthday party for my mother-in-law two days prior, complete with a decorated cake I had spent hours making and a crowded room of family members. I had used too much precious energy on that day, so it was no surprise that rest was needed on the next. I've found that when I overspend my energy account, it has to be repaid.

Looking over my plants, I decided to use a wagon to carry them down the long, steep hill to our meadow. Saving energy where I can is important when I am tackling a big project. I filled the wagon and started down the hill. The invigorating scent of the ponderosa pines along the way energized me. Being surrounded by nature is one of my favourite ways to nurture my wellbeing.

I retrieved my gardening tools from the shed and started digging. It felt good to be active and productive. After planting the raspberry canes and blueberry bushes, I stopped to assess my energy. Time for a break! To stay functional, I knew that I needed to pay close attention to my body and listen to its cues.

Trudging back up the hill with the wagon, I paused to enjoy my surroundings. I felt a bit out of breath, so the brief rest helped with that. My legs felt tired, but I made sure to focus on the beauty around me and reassured myself that it was normal to feel fatigued. Over-focusing on unpleasant sensations can sometimes trigger symptoms. When I started up the hill again, I coached myself through the steps: 'Just take four more steps. I think I can do four more. I'm doing great! 1, 2, 3, 4.' Taking my mind off of the fatigue by counting kept my brain from overreacting to normal sensations of weakness.

After a restorative break for lunch, I gathered the rest of the trees in the wagon and headed back down the hill. I dug a shallow trench for the trees' temporary home until the temperatures warmed up. Nestling them in the ground, I felt a sense of pride that I was able to accomplish such a huge task.

It wouldn't have been possible to do something like this a few years ago. My FND had overtaken my life and function back then. I wasn't able to walk, much less climb hills and dig trenches.

My FND began over 20 years ago. Since that time, I had run the gamut of symptoms, starting with seizures, then moving on to walking difficulties, episodes of uncontrollable movements, and problems with speech. I had enjoyed a relatively symptom-free period of seven years, then symptoms returned with a vengeance around the time that my mother was diagnosed with dementia. At that time, it was thought that I perhaps shared my mother's rare dementia diagnosis.

My symptoms advanced rapidly. My mobility deteriorated to the point that a wheelchair was necessary. My most distressing symptom was my loss of speech. It was so frustrating to be unable to communicate even basic needs. I felt trapped in my body, and no one could tell me what to do about it. The frustration was almost unbearable. I moved into an assisted living facility so that I could receive the full-time care that I needed.

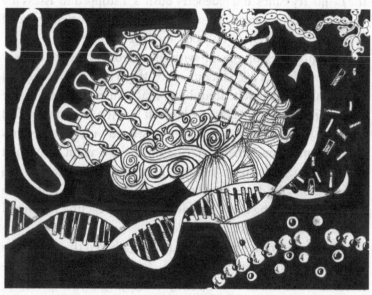

'Unravelling' expresses my confusion about what was happening with my brain and my life when my diagnosis didn't make sense to me

After about five years with this new diagnosis, my doctors decided that my symptoms were better explained by FND. When I was told that my increased symptoms were most likely functional, I knew I was faced with a choice. I could continue to deny my diagnosis, or I could face it head-on and try to get better. There was no help or support from my doctors, but thankfully the internet had information that was invaluable. Resources from FND Hope and neurosymptoms.org reassured me that I wasn't alone, and I wasn't crazy. I began to experiment with different techniques to help my brain to function better.

I wish I could say that I no longer have FND, but I'm thankful that at least I now know how to manage my symptoms. Listening to my body, pacing my activity, mindfulness, time in nature, creativity, helpful self-talk, healthy habits – these are all practices that have changed my function for the better. Not every day is a busy, productive day filled with challenging tasks, but finding that fragile balance between work and rest has helped me to create a life I love.

Like my garden and orchard, a healthy environment and nurturance help me to flourish. My health is my top priority now. It takes persistence to keep my symptoms under control, but the reward of a productive, satisfying life is totally worth it.

36

A Poem: FND Sucks

Female, 54 years old, Canada

FUNCTIONAL MOVEMENT DISORDER

Life was good before I got sick
No depression at all not even a hint
Trying hard as I can with all of my might
I don't want to lose this vicious fight

My children are grown but still want their mom
I want to be there for them healthy and strong
I want to live for myself and for my girls
Want to see them get older with wrinkles and pearls

There is no magic potion or no magic pill
There are limited treatments to try and get well
My brain and body are both perplexed
With a disorder that medicine leaves out on the fence

So what can I do when I've tried all there is
And nothing is working to fix what it is

It needs research and treatment of its own accord
How I wish the doctors would just get on board

My quality of life is worse than the pits
I want to live my life and not just exist

A Poem: Like a Phoenix

Female, 30 years old, UK

FND

FND where do I end, and you begin?
We feel like one as you writhe beneath my fiery burning skin.
I hate that you are with me
The sickly stand-off we are in
You are the Hyde to my Jekyll
It takes more from me to face you
In each sweat-soaked, boiling battle
Why must you leave me here in this bed
And make fireworks rip through my pounding head?
You've taken so much life from me
Even the pleasure of a hug
You make me lay awake at night
As my skin crawls with phantom bugs.
But don't think you'll ever beat me
For I'll win this fierce game.
You think you'll break me, but you can't
Like a Phoenix I'll thrive in flames

The Journey to Diagnosis

Female, 29 years old, Australia

FUNCTIONAL SEIZURES

The small, grey room is dimly lit, amplifying the whirr and sigh of the machines.

The examiner hovers, fingertips poised as if to give me a scalp massage. 'So, what brings you here, Amelia [pseudonym]?' he asks, patiently, routinely.

'Uh...' I gesture to the wires, accidentally bumping one of the electrodes.

'Careful.' His breath on my neck makes me squirm. 'Let's get you on the bed.'

A glimmer of warmth as a starched pillow is positioned beneath my Medusa head. *Don't get too comfortable.* I recall the receptionist's warning. Darkness fills the void.

A disembodied voice. 'Keep talking, Amelia.'

In the shower. Late November. A string of hot, sleepless nights. It starts with a vision. A daydream I can't switch off. Beneath the warm cocoon of cascading water, my surroundings stretch and detach. I am not in my own skin anymore. Suddenly, whoosh – an aircraft losing altitude. Abstract images surge into my head like a suspicious download. Snatches of sound. Laughter drips from the white-tiled walls. Searing pain stretches across my head, tightening like a torture device. Then comes the déjà vu, waves of nausea, as if I've been walloped in the guts. I am still staring at the wall when my partner, Toby [pseudonym], rushes in, asking why I've let the water run cold for 45 minutes. I try to respond, but my tongue has lost its will. He turns off the exhausted taps, and carries me to bed where I remain, still and mute, until morning wipes the slate clean.

Blinking myself back to the grey room, I wait for the examiner to interject, like doctors usually do. 'Oh, a panic attack? Anxiety? Depression? Suicidal ideation? Here's a script, we've got a pill for that.' But he is silent, so I continue.

Another day, another waiting room. Seventy-two hours since my last episode. I still can't form words properly. I tell the doctor how I couldn't find my way home, banging on the door of the wrong apartment...and the strange hours that followed, now glimpses through frosted glass. How trips to the supermarket end in panic because my god, everything is so damn bright. Lights pulse, colours bleed, the world warps. How Toby prepared green Thai curry, my favourite, but all I could taste was chalk, and in place of pak choi and brown rice were entrails and writhing maggots. How, in the midst of these turns, I am repulsed by human touch – and yet pulled further into myself.

The doctor returns to his default posture, staring at his computer, keys clacking. 'So, what's the problem?'

Steady. Breathe. 'I need...an MRI referral.'

'No referral. MRI is private, you pay.'

'...and the medical certificate?'

'You can work just fine. If you count writing as a "job".'

He then proceeds to point out, humourlessly, that Centrelink [service for people receiving benefit payments] is down the road. I lose my nerve and walk out.

The MRI is normal, but further tests are needed.

At home, I do what any self-respecting millennial would do: I google it. EEG. Uh-lek-trow-en-sef-uh-luh-gram. I roll each syllable on my tongue and scroll the 'helpful' algorithmic questions Google posits: Is an EEG painful? Will it trigger a seizure? Statistically, how likely is electrocution?

Back in the grey room, my body is bathed in a soft glow.

'So, that's it?' I sit up, forgetting the tentacles gripping my cranium.

'Not quite. Now I want you to hyperventilate.'

Whatever it takes to get those brainwaves jiving... I inhale, sounding like the foot pump Dad uses to inflate our camping beds. In and out. The motion sets off internal alarm bells. The image of a runaway Frankenstein bride, trailing wires and sparking electrodes, unnerves me. But before I can escape, an apparatus is positioned over my face.

'Lie back and close your eyes.' *Don't get too comfortable.*

I grip the bed rail as pulses of light flare. My brain and body unclasp... I am caught between silent submission and throes of feverish shaking. As I spill from the confines of my malfunctioning body, blotchy hands secure a compression band. Cold stethoscope to my chest. Pocket torch in my eyes. 'Slight anisocoria [unequal pupil size]. Heart rate 130. Blood pressure 140 over 90. Keep her in for ten.'

Fear claws under my skin. Only tears make my inner world known.

A clipboard dangles. 'Sign here and you're good to go.'

Good to go? Have I overstayed my welcome at a face-painting stall? I scribble something that resembles my name and slip, wraith-like, from the room.

Outside, the day lies before me like a wasteland.

Two weeks later, I get the call. The neurologist has a kind smile and too-white teeth. I want to trust him. But I also want him to trust me.

'So, Amelia, what brings you here today?' This question, I realize, is a technique.

On my lap is a dossier of journal articles and a book, *Hysteria*, by Katerina Bryant. I explain that Katerina's experience is not unlike my own. In fact, the parallels are unnerving. 'Katerina has functional neurological disorder or FND, which falls in the grey area between psychiatry and neurology.'

He nods at the diagnosis I am handing him on a manila platter. 'So, you identify as someone with this disorder?'

I hold his gaze for longer than we both feel comfortable.

'Amelia, we are on your side. We want to fix this.'

On his desk is my case file: 'MRI and EEG normal. Working diagnosis: FND.' Scrawled beneath is: *Neurologist? Psychiatrist?*

But my specialist doesn't write any referrals. He jots down a website he says will be useful for 'grouping my symptoms' and then discharges me with a patient, routine smile.

As I walk out, it occurs to me that this is no longer a constellation of symptoms but a potent, fully formed thing. I want to care for it. I have a responsibility. I have a *response ability*. I pat the top of my head, and say: 'Brain, we have work to do.'

Outside, the day stretches before me like a wonderland.

Reference

Bryant, K. (2020). *Hysteria: A memoir of illness, strength and women's stories throughout history*. Montgomery, AL: NewSouth Publishing.

39

Resilience

Female, 47 years old, UK

FUNCTIONAL SEIZURES

I was obviously concerned while in hospital struggling to mobilize and having constant seizure episodes. The consultant asked me if I had ever had depression and I answered 'no'. They asked about my family life. I felt as if he thought it was a psychological issue. The day after my MRI scan results were clear, the consultant just said, 'Home tomorrow. I deal with facts and numbers and yours are all okay.' I fully understood what he meant (it was all in my head and there was nothing really wrong). Even though I wasn't walking very well and having constant seizure episodes, I was so happy to go home to my family who love me.

I felt let down by the hospital and the staff. I was unable to speak properly so couldn't explain myself very well and had no visitors due to Covid-19 infection control restrictions. Once home, I looked at my discharge letter and my diagnosis. I looked up the website I was given, and it was as if it was written for me. I could not believe it, all my symptoms mirrored what the website said. I was dragging my right leg, intermittent paralysis, extreme fatigue and severe speech issues. I joined a forum on Facebook and quickly learned that I needed to help myself as this condition is not very well understood. I looked at YouTube videos of people having therapy and realized what I was doing wrong. I had to distract myself. I made good progress and even managed to get back to work. I printed information off for my boss and work colleagues to educate them and to ignore my seizure-like episodes.

It's been hard and I keep having two steps forward and three back. I'm learning what triggers the episodes. The sun is a trigger. I have warning signs, such as I salivate from my mouth. I am still learning and trying to stay positive.

FND is real, it is not made up; the symptoms are bizarre. I never know if I can walk properly every single time I get up from my chair. I am strong and a fighter and it is that resilience and strong mindset that have helped me keep going with no support from any medical professional, as I have not had any follow-up to date.

40

Lessons in Hope: What FND Means to Me

Female, 52 years old, UK

FUNCTIONAL SEIZURES

In my forties, I had a near-death accident that exacerbated my dissociative (functional) seizures to a life-threatening level. At their worst, I had seven a day, in the middle of crossroads, at the edge of train platforms and in supermarket queues. At this time, to protect my head, I started wearing a rugby helmet decorated with butterfly stickers – no one batted an eyelid as everyone knows how eccentric English people can be!

Since then, I've made a dramatic recovery. Over the last two years I've led a Covid-19 communications team, entailing long hours and tight deadlines. What helped? A determination to understand my condition, a wholehearted engagement with CBT and a deep conviction to never let a fear of falling rule my life.

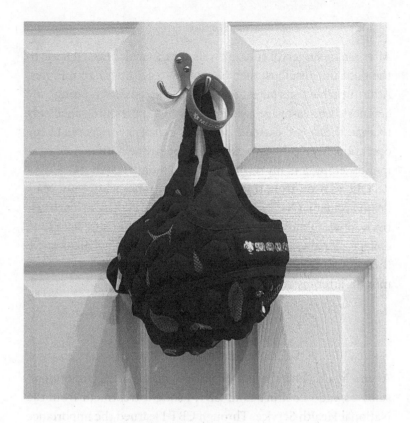

My 31-year diagnostic journey

Teens

First seizure: crumpled to the floor as if I'd had a dead faint. I continued collapsing once a year, at parties where I was the centre of attention, often crying with laughter.

Twenties

Diagnosed with a 'petit mal' (epilepsy) triggered by extreme happiness. Who knew it was possible to be 'too happy for your own good'? By then I'd learned to avoid seizures by calming down quickly when my head felt as if it was being crushed in a vice.

Forties

After major surgery, I couldn't walk for three months. I'd fizzle to the floor unconscious, then be unable to get up for 20 minutes. After tilt table tests [a test to examine the cause of fainting], my diagnosis was vasovagal syncope (low blood pressure), an allergy to anaesthesia and extreme hormone deficiency triggered by my operation. My weakness was resolved by strong hormone replacement therapy, and my seizures stopped months later.

One year on from this, I had a major relapse after my near-death accident. Over the next eight months, I was tested exhaustively for brain tumours, heart problems, blood pressure issues and epilepsy. Finally, a neuropsychiatrist confirmed I had dissociative (functional) seizures and recommended CBT, which I started ten months after my accident.

Discovering what works

As my health insurance didn't cover dissociative (functional) seizures and I couldn't fund CBT, I sought treatment from the National Health Service. Through CBT I learned the importance of recognizing my triggers, identifying pre-seizure symptoms, and techniques for seizure 'management'.

My CBT expert was unsurprised by my diagnosis, given how accident prone I am. I've sustained multiple concussions that rendered me unconscious through playing different sports, and I've had life-threatening experiences such as sustaining third-degree burns and getting lost in a temperate rainforest where I was in danger from wild animals.

Every week for seven months, I completed 'homework' and carefully navigated the three-hour round trip to the hospital alone. The latter felt like dicing with death, with seizures happening on the journey there or back. Sometimes, I would sit in the waiting room for two hours before attempting the trip home, because CBT had prompted bad seizures.

By the time I was discharged, I'd learned to manage my seizures through:

- distraction techniques – counting anything
- regulating my body temperature
- pacing myself, prioritizing down-time
- daily meditation and sport
- sleeping for seven hours
- wearing noise-cancelling headphones
- processing anger and frustration.

Within two weeks, my mother died suddenly. I was devastated. Challenging as it was, the techniques helped and I coped: my fabulous CBT expert provided me with practical advice on how to handle the funeral.

Battling to return to work

Initially, after my near-death accident, work was very understanding. On my first return, I collapsed and became unconscious four times in one hour. My sympathetic manager sent me home. Six months later, everyone's patience had worn thin. Every month I was being investigated for another illness and it all seemed mad to me too!

After one year, I asked to return to the office, despite my continued seizures. To facilitate this the health and safety officer (HSO) met me, my neuropsychiatrist and CBT expert. During this meeting, a heated debate broke out about whether I was disabled. I felt blindsided by the discussion; 'disabled' was not a label I wanted to wear, as I feared it would be career-limiting. Everyone assured me that this would provide me with 'protection' in the workplace – and I now know it does. But at the time, I was so angry it triggered a seizure that frightened the HSO.

Subsequently, I was only permitted to return to the office after completing an occupational health assessment. It took weeks to arrange, and I was unprepared for the experience. Unnervingly, it was undertaken at my home by an occupational health adviser, with my manager present.

The adviser confessed he'd never heard of my condition, nor read the information I had sent him. He questioned me in detail about my medical history, in front of my manager; it felt highly intrusive and irrelevant. Afterwards, I faced several quick-fire tests designed for those two levels above my post. It was stressful, and towards the end I became so dizzy and tearful that we had to stop for five minutes. After the three-hour session, I could barely walk.

Despite my good test results, I spent two months battling to get the adviser's recommendations changed. Thankfully, my neuropsychiatrist wrote explaining I wasn't 'brain damaged', the tests were inappropriate, and the stipulation that I complete a three-month phased return into the office or face demotion was superfluous. This helped my manager understand more about my condition and together we agreed a plan for my return.

The changes at work were minimal but important. They were easy to adopt and included:

- wearing a medical alert bracelet
- raising team awareness
- working from home several days a week
- avoiding rush hour
- using quiet-rooms and noise-cancelling headphones
- negotiating evacuation procedures.

Not letting fear of falling rule my life

Discovering what FND means for me has taken time and I'm still learning. I've never let those three letters define me, nor have I let a fear of falling hold me back. It hasn't been easy but now people who don't know about my seizures just see me having a high-powered job and an active social life.

FND isn't just a diagnosis or a stigmatic label: it's part of my life. Without determination though, it can expand until there's no difference between the definition of FND and the definition of you. With effort, you can manage it, so that you (and it) know its place. Living with FND is never boring; it's laced with shots of black humour and can be debilitating, challenging and wholly inexplicable. But it's never, ever, bigger than you.

41

Primum Non Nocere (First, Do No Harm): A Neurologist's Story

Neurologist and researcher, seven years'
experience of working with FND, UK

Early experiences tend to mark us most. Matt [pseudonym] was one of the first patients with FND that I met, yet years later he remains vividly in my mind and exemplifies many aspects I have repeatedly witnessed.

Matt had a long history of migraines, for which he received numerous treatments. At the age of 50, anti-dopaminergic anti-nausea medication led to a transient oculogyric crisis, a known acute side effect involving involuntary upward deviation of the eyes. Six months later, he developed more severe intermittent, abnormal movements of his legs. Following a hospitalization and FND diagnosis, the abnormal eye movements gradually disappeared, but he continued to experience intermittent abnormal leg movements.

After years of follow-up, Matt was hospitalized for a second opinion on his wish to undergo deep brain stimulation (DBS). DBS is a surgical intervention in which electrodes are implanted in a specific part of the brain, allowing modulation with effective inactivation of that brain area. This is very effective for many movement disorders, including Parkinson's disease, tremor and tardive dystonia, which is abnormal posturing induced by long-term anti-dopaminergic medication, the diagnosis Matt erroneously believed he had. The consultant explained that he had FND and that DBS was not an appropriate treatment. One evening, I spent several hours trying to explain the diagnosis, and that psychological therapy was the way forward, not DBS. At the time, psychotherapy was the only available FND treatment. We weren't yet aware of FND experts, specialized physiotherapy or other treatments. I felt nervous, which I hardly ever did talking to patients. I realized that it was because my explanations made very little sense to me. Now, after years of clinical and research experience, I am very comfortable explaining the diagnosis as I can stand by it. I am convinced that patients can sense that and that this in itself has a therapeutic effect. Despite my lack of experience at the time, Matt was surprisingly receptive, and I remember feeling very optimistic when leaving late in the evening. The next morning, however, his wife was by his side, adamantly and angrily opposing the diagnosis, and Matt followed her. I felt disheartened and powerless.

Several years later, I heard from a colleague at another hospital that Matt had later asked them for DBS, which was refused. To our major surprise, DBS was subsequently performed privately in North America. It initially led to major improvement, but it was only short-lived, and had no long-term benefit.

Matt exemplifies many common aspects: an initial triggering event such as medication side effects; difficulties explaining the diagnosis by non-experienced physicians; lack of appropriate FND treatments due to lack of expertise; anger and strong opposition to the diagnosis; negative interference by family members; and doctor-shopping out of desperation. Nevertheless, the standout ones, in my opinion, are the concept of first, do no harm, *primum non nocere*, and the placebo effect with its slippery slope.

The ancient principle 'first, do no harm' appears obvious but can be opposed by doctors' and patients' wishes or impulses to do something. How can we 'do nothing' if the patient is suffering? However, 'doing something', such as giving medication or interventions without clear indications may cause more harm than good.

The neurosurgeon performing Matt's DBS might have believed his erroneous self-diagnosis or felt that doing something was better than leaving him the way he was. However, DBS is a major neuro-surgical intervention which could have led to severe complications. Matt was fortunate that there were no direct complications, but it nevertheless cost him tens of thousands of pounds, lost time, physical stress and emotional turmoil. Furthermore, the implanted metalwork prevents him from having MRI scans outside specialist centres. The brain surgery clearly did more harm than good.

This makes me think of cases of crowdfunding for treatments that are unavailable via standard health services. In general, there is a good reason why they are not recommended for a par-ticular person, and going against the expertise can have serious consequences.

Initially, Matt's abnormal movements improved, which, in all likelihood, was due to a placebo effect. It is well-known that people with FND can experience major 'miracle-like' placebo effects, but, as in Matt's case, these often don't last long. Studies have shown that people with FND are not more susceptible to placebos as such, but if they do have a placebo effect, the degree can be much larger than in people with non-functional conditions. In a person with, say, functional leg weakness symptoms, there is no structural damage, so there is no physical limit to the extent to which the placebo effect can act. In a person with leg weakness due to a spinal injury, the damage to the spine will set a clear boundary to any placebo effect.

Given that dramatic placebo effects can occasionally occur in FND, some might argue that it is cruel not to try. The main argu-ments against it stem from the concept of *primum non nocere*; the fact that placebo treatments can cause harm. They might involve lying to the patient, pretending that it is a drug or intervention that helps their condition, when in fact there is no evidence for it and the intention is purely a placebo effect. This could destroy the doctor-patient relationship with dire consequences of lack of trust in the long term. Additionally, there is the slippery slope of placebo treatments. Their effects, as in Matt's case, are often short-lived and it is well known that the more drastic the procedure, the stronger the placebo effect. One could therefore fall into a vicious spiral of more and more risky procedures being performed.

Thankfully, I have never seen another person with FND undergoing unnecessary brain surgery. With improved knowledge, cases such as Matt's are hopefully becoming rarer as better explanations help people understand their diagnosis, and improved access to the right treatments replace inappropriate ones or the lack thereof.

42

I am Safe

Female, 63 years old, US

FUNCTIONAL SEIZURES

'I am safe.' Three simple words. One hundred and eight times. Twenty-one days. This practice is the last piece of the puzzle that gets me through FND. My journey began over two years ago, while I was alone in our basement. My right side shook. I couldn't speak, I was weak, disoriented and scared I was having a stroke. After it stopped, I got up to the first floor yelling 'Help!' It was my first non-epileptic (functional) seizure (NES). Over a week and 500 NES later, the neurologist diagnosed me with FND. She told me some people have one episode and never have another; FND puts you in a constant state of fight or flight and when triggered with a perceived threat, the brain misfires into an NES. To help FND, she said I had to deal with stress and calm my nervous system. Although she didn't recommend alternative medicine, this is my story of how I use many alternative healing modalities to move beyond FND's debilitating grip.

Because of constant NES, I couldn't do yoga or acupuncture but thought maybe reiki would work. At my first treatment, I lay on a table while the reiki master scanned each of my seven chakras; all were closed. As one chakra (energy centre) was opened, my body felt so heavy, as if I couldn't move and was melting into the table. Afterwards, I felt better, calmer, more together. As I tracked the seizures during the following days, I realized the full impact – fewer NES! After just five weekly treatments, I went from having 60 seizures a day to just one, usually while falling asleep. Since reiki dramatically reduced the frequency of my seizures, it gave me hope that my life could be more than just enduring repetitive NES. Not having seizures during the day gave me time to analyse my situation. I knew my subconscious was still in turmoil because of the night-time NES. With each one, I felt the hypnotic tug and swirl of the NES pulling me into nothingness. Plus, I was very distracted and scattered, as exhibited by my memory, speech and cognitive issues. It felt as if I was an observer of my own life, not really living it. I realized these symptoms described a lack of a mind-body-spirit connection.

I used several practices to rebuild my mind-body-spirit connection. The slow, intentional movement of beginner yoga and the balance poses of Ghosh yoga nudged me back into my body. Deep breathing work, inspirational readings, spiritual music and journalling helped me get in touch with my spirit. Grounding improved my scattered thoughts and was easy to do. I just sat outside, especially barefoot, letting the earth do its natural electromagnetic energy exchange, and I slept with a weighted blanket. Cross-body techniques like alternate nostril breathing could integrate the right and left hemispheres of the brain, but I was too fatigued to practise it. Instead, I made figure of eights with my hands or feet to facilitate integration. Over time, I felt the strengthening of my mind-body-spirit connection and as a result, I only had a seizure about twice a month.

Unfortunately, when Covid-19 hit, I stopped doing yoga and my NES changed into something which mimicked a 'grand mal' or epileptic seizure: unconscious, foaming at the mouth, full body rigidity. Each of these seizures warranted a trip to the ER for blood work, IV fluids and several hours under observation until I regained coherence. Desperate for answers, I compared my lab results, combed through my anatomy and physiology textbook and researched my FND symptoms. Unable to figure out what to do, I saw a naturopathic doctor. Lab results from eight vials of blood and a hair sample showed deficiencies in potassium, iodine, serine and cysteine and low levels of other nutrients necessary for brain health and energy. If I corrected these out-of-range results with supplements, perhaps my body could maintain homeostasis on its own. After starting, I went three months without a seizure! Plus, my fatigue was lessening and my cognition was improving. Having more energy and the ability to think clearly made me want to resume doing more 'normal' things, but I was afraid. Sometimes I feel the 'F' in FND should stand for fear rather than functional. It was pervasive throughout my experience. I was afraid of the dark, being alone, leaving my yard, not remembering, speaking incorrectly, or experiencing one of my NES triggers (flashing lights, loud noises, tripping). These irrational fears did not exist prior to FND.

I found the answer to conquer my fears in *Switch on Your Brain* by Dr Caroline Leaf. Her book explains how the brain creates a thought, a pattern, a memory, and how to use this natural process to create a positive neural response in just 21 days. Using this process, I examined my feelings and thoughts and everything pointed to fear. For me, the opposite of fear was safety and so my first active reach became, 'I am safe.' Every morning, I said, 'I am safe' for each bead on my mala and this practice created a new positive neural response. If uneasiness arose, 'I am safe' popped into my head and calmed my inner storm. The piece of me who drove, travelled, and lived, was coming back. Repeating 'I am safe' every day rebuilt my confidence. In essence, the neurologist who diagnosed me thought my FND was stress induced and I began a fascinating exploration of alternative ways to relieve stress and calm my nervous system. I am grateful the neurologist gave me hope that FND need not overtake my life. If you are stuck with the same or worsening FND symptoms, perhaps some of these alternative healing modalities might work for you. What have you got to lose? Maybe FND.

Reference

Leaf, C. (2013). *Switch on Your Brain. Grand Rapids, MI: Baker Books.*

43

Emotional Pain

Specialist psychotherapist, eight years'
experience of working with FND, UK

I was reflecting on what I wanted to say about working with patients with FND and found myself wanting to think about what is happening in different ways. Often when I think about FND with a very particular and extremely troubling physical presentation, I tend to try to understand the science. What is causing this? How can I measure it? What can I do about it? This cause-and-effect model is important and helpful; however, we are human beings and there is room for a more nuanced way of thinking about this condition. The philosophical tradition is almost entirely excluded from academic writing about FND. The enlightenment tradition with rationalism and science almost completely dominates. Both ways of understanding the world are valid; each person must choose what to believe, but I'm struck by how dominant the scientific and reductive tradition is in our culture. And perhaps this closes off ways of being which in turn leads to illness.

The individual narrative gives a greater richness that self-report questionnaires cannot provide, yet so much of what we think about FND comes from quantitative data. Thinking about the wider societal context of our patient's experience is also important. Given the wide variety of presenting issues and circumstances that our patients have, it is unlikely that we will get an overarching understanding that is relevant to all the people we see. However, the themes are also very interesting to notice.

I am drawn to quoting James Hillman, a Jungian psychotherapist, who wrote eloquently about the soul, and I think his way of thinking reflects how rational, scientific ways of approaching people and the world is only one aspect of who we are.

> ...aggression, violence, power; sadism – aren't shadows at all; that's the whole western ego! Go ahead, get ahead, do it. It's only what that breaks down, when depression comes in, and you can't get up and do it. When impotence happens and you can't get on with it. When you feel beaten, oppressed, knocked back....then something moves and you begin to feel yourself as soul. (Hillman, 1998, p.11)

He goes on to say:

> The culture expects one to be manic: hyperactive, spend and consume and waste, be very verbal, flow of ideas, don't stay too long with anything – the fear of being boring – and we lose the sense of sadness. (Hillman, 1998, p.13)

Our culture encourages a way of being which rewards activity and action. What does this do to other aspects of how we are in the world? What does it mean to have your ability to move as a result of FND affected in this context?

I was reminded of this recently with a patient who has had a deep and profound experience of psychotherapy for his FND symptoms. It was our last (20th) session and he had found during the week prior to our 19th session that his legs were giving way again and he was unable to walk. I gently wondered if he might be feeling sad about our work coming to an end. He had reflected on this over the week and said that he realized it was stupid and not rational to be sad about therapy ending as he always knew it would end. When he acknowledged and valued his actual feelings over the week, he found he had no symptoms and was able to walk with no problems. He was quite wry about this and said that having to be aware of and in contact with his many and varied feelings was difficult and in some ways the symptoms were easier to deal with. His story was one of the most pronounced examples of putting other people before oneself; the term 'unmitigated communion' is used to describe this. His parents had not valued his sensitivity and empathic nature and had encouraged him to take up boxing and enter the army. He had then been in an abusive relationship for many years. He had retreated to a place where he did not feel anything and initially said he was happy and had no issues. His journey through therapy was to start to connect his experience of his life with the wall he had created around himself, which meant that he felt little and was separated from everything and everyone. It was an uncomfortable process for him where the physical symptoms often seemed preferable to the depth of feelings that he kept at bay.

> In the arts you don't use opposites. You may say there are strong contrasts in a painting... I don't think about conscious versus unconscious...or passivity versus activity; I try to stick with what is presented. (Hillman, 1998, p.14)

This approach does not mean that symptoms and the very real physical struggles that people experience do not matter, but that the way we respond to them is different. Often clinicians can get caught in what objectively happened for a patient: were they close to dying or not in this medical emergency? This, I think, misses the point, the way the medical event appeared to the patient, the meaning, the lack of control, the resonances with other experiences in their life might be more important in how their recovery unfolds. Many patients with FND seem to have a limited capacity to express themselves emotionally and yet they have a huge ability to impact us as practitioners emotionally, whether it is to roll our eyes at the exaggeration or feel pulled to try to sort out their complex and difficult lives. I like Hillman's work because it reminds me to be with what is presented and to be curious about it without being pulled to try to cure the other. There is something very powerful about being with another person without trying to fix them. Perhaps when we think about FND we could think about emotional pain unexpressed. The body is saying what the conscious mind is trying to ignore.

> The pathology is the place that keeps the person in the soul, that torment, that twist that you can't simply be naive, you can't simply go along in a natural way, that there's something broken, twisted, hurting, that forces constant reflection... If you come at pathology from a psychological perspective, then you're dealing with pathology in terms of the soul's way of working on itself. (Hillman, 1998, p.23)

Reference

Hillman, J. (1998). *Inter Views: Conversations with Laura Pozzo on Psychotherapy, Biography, Love, Soul, Dreams, Work, Imagination, and the State of the Culture*. Thompson, CT: Spring Publications.

44

Motherhood and FND

Female, 39 years old, US

FUNCTIONAL MOVEMENT DISORDER

When I dreamed about the mother I'd eventually become, I always dreamed of lots of arts and crafts, creativity, hikes, the zoo, museums, being a sports mom, and cooking and baking with my kids. Doing fun activities together and creating beautiful, lasting memories from our experiences. Well, life didn't really turn out that way. Motherhood with FND looks more like extra cuddles, TV time, story time, short walks, occasional trips to the playground, and other activities where I can sit or lounge while doing them. The chronic fatigue, dystonia, gait issues, brain fog and sensory sensitivities (just to name a few of my many symptoms) heavily limit my physical abilities.

When I first became pregnant nine years ago, I had FND but was going into remission. About six months earlier, I came off a medication thought to have interacted with an antibiotic I was taking around the time of my trigger date. I had not been diagnosed with FND yet, and the doctors I saw thought I'd go into full recovery. In the three years that followed, I was in remission, worked full time, had mild symptoms mostly at night, and delivered two babies. Six weeks after I gave birth to my second child, I started to relapse. Since I didn't have a diagnosis, I didn't know what I needed to do to take care of my body, and I pushed it to its extreme. This had devastating consequences, and it became the most challenging year of my life.

A year later and a trip to the hospital, I was finally diagnosed with FND, six and a half years after my FND journey began. My children were still very young at this point, and they have never known me as a well mom. For this, I am grateful. I know how hard it was for me to grieve for my well self, and I'm glad they've never had to grieve for their well mother.

Motherhood with FND comes with its unique challenges. I can no longer cook, so if my husband is out during dinner time it's either leftovers or sandwiches. Maybe a quesadilla if I'm having a good day. Playdates have to be scheduled around my rests, and I can rarely do two activities in one weekend. If I do, I know I'll need extra rest afterwards, usually on a Monday. At times, it's been a struggle to see my kids disappointed because we can't do an activity due to my FND symptoms. They now know that while we can't do it today or this week, we can usually plan for it in the future. This doesn't always go over well with younger kids, but they have started to grasp the concept now that they are in elementary school. But they are also learning things that I was never taught growing up, like how to relax and be okay with doing nothing. We actually have what we call lazy Sundays where we pretty much do nothing because it's a rest day for me and my husband. And I know they certainly get more hugs, kisses and cuddle time from me than they would have if I was a well mom.

I was always on the go as a kid. That's how I would have run my house, too, if I had never got FND because, honestly, I didn't know how to live a balanced life and societal expectations ruled my life. In the past, I have been plagued with extreme guilt thinking I wasn't a good enough mom because I live with FND. It took grieving the mother I wanted to be to accept the mother I actually am. The grieving process and practising self-compassion helped me realize that, in reality, I'm doing pretty well at being a mom, and I am good enough just as I am.

One mindset shift I try to live by is to focus on the things I can do. I can touch base with my children after school and see how they are doing and feeling. I can give them infinite hugs and cuddles. I can still laugh and be silly with them, and we can still make beautiful memories together, even if it's only from the couch in our living room.

45

FND and Competitive Sports

Neurologist, 30 years' experience
of working with FND, UK

David

All four corners of David's [pseudonym] wheelchair had been strapped firmly to the ground. He leaned back and turned his head, neck and back over to the right as far as he could, stabilizing himself with his left hand which was grabbing a pole cemented into the ground. As his head and shoulders spun round to the left, he extended his right arm and fired the metal ball he had been holding close to his ear away into a cloudless sky. They say that taking part is all that matters – but somehow, he knew that he had produced the shot put of his life and that he may have won a medal.

I am a neurologist. As I make diagnoses and propose treatments to those who have come to me asking for help, I rarely need to concern myself with the extent to which one cause of weakness may be less disabling or more variable than another. My patients do not usually compete with each other to establish who has the weaker legs. However, David was an exceptional patient.

It is one of the characteristic features of FND that its manifestations are 'inconsistent'. One way in which FND can be inconsistent is that weakness may be present in one particular situation but not in another. This could be one of the reasons why clinicians, family members and even those experiencing the condition may ask whether FND symptoms are deliberately produced.

Perhaps we are so suspicious because we have all used illness as an excuse in our own lives. FND may arouse particular suspicion because the diagnosis may be confirmed by a clinician's ability to demonstrate that a particular function (e.g., pushing an affected leg down into the bed) can be carried out 'automatically' (e.g., when the good leg is being lifted off the bed) but not when the patient is asked to push the 'bad' leg down. This suspicion persists despite the fact that the brain activation triggered when a person with FND is told to move a paralysed limb differs from that seen in someone pretending not to be able to move the limb. Put simply, the motor networks of those pretending to be weak show little activity when they are asked to move but don't. In contrast, those with FND activate their movement networks much like people without paralysis who are able to carry out the movement. However, in addition, those with FND activate other areas in the brain. This 'excess' brain activity seems to get in the way of instructions from the brain getting through to the muscles. These studies suggest functional weakness is not caused by pretending – or not trying hard enough. If anything, people with FND are trying too hard.

But let me tell you more about David. He had been a bit of a loner at school although he had always taken great care of his body. He felt respected by the other body builders in his gym. David's life changed dramatically when he was involved in an accident at work when he was 22. He lost his balance while carrying building materials up a ladder and ended up two floors below with his right temple impaled on a piece of scaffolding.

David only regained consciousness in hospital after the front of his right temporal lobe and fragments of his skull bone had been surgically removed. At first, David seemed to recover remarkably well. He had no problems with arm or leg movements. Unfortunately, a week after his accident, David developed signs of a wound infection. Despite intensive treatment with antibiotics, he had to undergo more surgery to remove further fragments of his skull bone.

Six months after his initial discharge David was readmitted for a planned insertion of a titanium plate that was designed to close the hole in his skull which the accident and his earlier surgeries had left. The operation went as planned. However, as David was coming round from the anaesthetic his whole body went into a seizure. The seizure activity did not stop when the anaesthetist administered two doses of medication. I was asked to see him urgently and recognized that the seizure movements were irregular and not like those of an epileptic seizure. His eyes were closed. I diagnosed a dissociative seizure, told everyone to step back and to allow me to talk to David. As I addressed him by his name, told him that the operation had gone well and that he was now in the recovery area, the seizure movements began to settle. However, when he had come round from the seizure, he was unable to move his legs.

The next five years were a dark period of David's life. He stopped looking after his body and became depressed. I had come to the conclusion that his leg weakness and his inability to sit unaided were a manifestation of FND. MRI scans of his brain and spine showed that the movement centres and motor pathways of his nervous system had not been injured in the accident or operations. Unfortunately, physiotherapy did not produce any sustained improvements. David had a few appointments with a psychotherapist but then stopped going because he was very uncomfortable talking to a stranger about things which he considered private.

However, David's life turned round completely after he watched the Invictus Games, an athletics competition for disabled soldiers. He was fired up by the idea that people in wheelchairs could get involved in sports. The next morning, he got in touch with his local athletics team. They had experience with disabled sports and invited David to come along.

David discovered his talent for wheelchair shot-putting. He worked hard to build up his upper body strength and improve his technique. His depression was a thing of the past. Within 12 months David was winning international competitions. Before long he had secured a place on his national Paralympics team.

However, just as he was entering the final training for the Paralympics he received a letter from the team physician: the diagnosis of FND implied that David had too much voluntary control over his movements to qualify for the Paralympics. In order to ensure that he met the latest rules defining medical conditions allowing athletes to participate in the Paralympics, David would need a further medical assessment and a different diagnosis.

At this point, a very disheartened David had a follow-up appointment with me. I had seen how the shot-putting had changed David's life completely and could imagine what might happen, if David could not compete in his sport anymore. David had been living with a significant disability for many years, which had resisted all of my previous treatment efforts. I could not believe that David had any voluntary control over his symptoms or that he was 'putting on' his weakness. What should I do?

I arranged another brain scan in the hope that the definite brain damage from David's injury might extend from his right temporal lobe to parts of his brain directly involved in motor control. However, the repeat brain scan showed no damage in David's motor areas or motor tracts. I would have to rely on words alone to recast David's functional weakness in terms that might convince his team physician and the Paralympic medical advisers. I wrote them a letter describing the scan findings and arguing that the brain defect in the right temporal region was likely to be contributing to disturbance of brain networks relevant to motor control and causing 'ideomotor apraxia' – that is, a malfunction due to the disconnection of the 'idea' and 'movement' areas of the brain. While avoiding the words 'functional disorder', this seemed to be an honest description of our current understanding of FND. Having sent this letter, I did not hear from David for several months. Then came the announcement on national news:

David had won the silver medal in shot put in the Paralympic Games!

I was very pleased for David and wrote him a letter to congratulate him on his huge achievement. It has been a huge joy to see how his sport has helped him to turn his life around. But I do wonder: May David's functional sitting balance have improved in the moment he was concentrating on his upper limbs? Nevertheless, I continue to think that I did the right thing writing my letter. David worked very hard to overcome a disability over which he has no control. Since his retirement as an active athlete, he has inspired many other disabled people to find a new meaning for their life through sport.

46

Functional Cognitive Symptoms: Insights from a Neuropsychologist

Clinical neuropsychologist, five years'
post-doctorate, with a total of eight years'
experience of working with FND, US

As a neuropsychologist, I frequently see patients with functional cognitive symptoms, which are sometimes isolated, sometimes part of another FND or somatic symptom disorder, part of a post-concussive syndrome or illness anxiety disorder (e.g., dementia worry). Occasionally, patients have been previously diagnosed with dementia or major neurocognitive disorder (due to medical conditions that were suspected at the time) based on the presence of cognitive impairment and evidence of impact on IADLs (instrumental activities of daily living). What may not have been clear to those providers is that the patients had pre-emptively left their jobs, stopped driving, or handed over responsibilities to a spouse after making a minor (but uncharacteristic) mistake or simply out of anticipatory anxiety that they would make a mistake, get lost and so on. Incorrect diagnoses like this have the potential to cause significant iatrogenic harm to the patient. Neuropsychologists are in many ways well positioned to differentiate between functional cognitive disorder (FCD) and mild cognitive impairment or dementia, yet this is hindered by the lack of recognition of FCD as a diagnosis in the *Diagnostic and Statistical Manual of Mental Disorders* or the *International Classification of Diseases*.

I often explain functional cognitive symptoms to patients in the following ways.

When patients describe or show evidence of short-term or working memory difficulties (e.g., losing their train of thought, forgetting why they walked into a room, or making absent-minded mistakes) in the absence of a neurological or neurodegenerative process, there are often other factors present that are 'taking up brain space'. Chronic pain, stressors, worrying, ruminating or any abnormal body sensations (tinnitus, gastrointestinal symptoms, etc.) all essentially act like open browser tabs on a computer. You don't have to consciously be thinking about them for them to consume finite working memory resources. Some medical/psychiatric conditions (e.g., cerebrovascular disease, chronic insomnia, attention deficit hyperactivity disorder) and medications may also limit the number of 'tabs' our brains can keep open at once. Eventually if you don't close them, the computer will freeze. This leads to a discussion about what 'tabs' may be open and has relevance for treatment planning. This analogy came from a meme that I absolutely can relate to: 'My brain has too many tabs open, four are frozen, and I can't figure out which one the music is coming from.'

Other times, on testing, patients will display maladaptive coping or compensatory strategies out of anticipatory anxiety, fear of failure, or strategies that they have learned to avoid having to rely on their memory. Sometimes this manifests as distraction or tuning out difficult-to-process information (like when someone who hates maths only hears the voice of Charlie Brown's teacher say, 'wah wah wah wah' in a maths class). Other times, patients may use a very elaborate rehearsal strategy to remember information on tests that should otherwise be a straightforward repetition task – anything from forming associations between the information to be remembered with various objects in the room, or visualizing the written characters of the letters, and so on. Whenever I suspect that something like this is happening, I ask what kind of strategy they are using and then make this a point to bring up in feedback if the strategy seems to actually inhibit, rather than enhance, their performance.

Sometimes people who use these elaborate memory compensatory strategies are a bit 'type A' or perfectionistic in some ways. I explain that there is a law of diminishing or negative returns with the complexity of the memory or organizational system being used. Usually, simple is better. Sometimes people start repeatedly checking and double checking for errors as a result of losing confidence in their memory and fearing memory loss or making errors. Again, too much of this may not only be unhealthy but can also cause more memory problems. This is similar to the concept of 'semantic satiation' where staring at or repeatedly saying a word for too long makes it seem to lose its meaning. Repeated checking can cause a similar phenomenon and actually increase uncertainty.

These are common features that I see among patients with functional cognitive symptoms, and I find that patients typically relate to these explanations well.

47

The FND Puzzle

Female, 50 years old, Canada

FUNCTIONAL MOVEMENT DISORDER

In my late thirties, I started having major cognitive issues, such as losing track of what I did five minutes ago, forgetting names of colleagues at work, trouble finding words and so on. After this went away, I started having severe irritable bowel syndrome, which lasted about six months. Shortly after my 39th birthday, I began limping on my right leg. It got so bad I ended up in a wheelchair. For six months, my knee was flexed at a 45-degree angle and I was only able to jump on my left leg.

Needless to say, the doctors were baffled. Physical cause was ruled out, and I was referred to a neuropsychiatrist. He diagnosed me with conversion disorder. On finding out that I was single and childless, the neuropsychiatrist told me that this fact has made me resentful, and my emotions converted into a physical symptom. I wasn't buying it altogether, but on the other hand, I really wanted my dystonia to be psychogenic, because this is the only type of dystonia that is potentially reversible.

He referred me to CBT and put me on some medication. I plunged myself into psychotherapy, digging into my past. It's true that I have a history of trauma. I was bullied at school, went through a war in my homeland, and was in an abusive relationship. However, I had dealt with those problems through psychotherapy even before my dystonia, which is why I was confused when they told me I suppressed my emotions.

FND has affected me in a big way. First, it's how the symptoms keep changing all the time. Just as when I think I'm getting better, I get worse again. And it wasn't just the intensity of symptoms changing. The type of dystonia kept changing; the right knee would buckle when I'd try to walk or stand; sometimes it would turn inward, sometimes outward when I walked, sometimes it would start jerking. It looked very weird to people, and I got stared at many times. It was hard not only putting up with such changeable symptoms, but also trying to explain my condition to others. Although I was very active before my dystonia, I could no longer walk, hike or socialize whenever I felt like it. Everything became a lot more complicated. Friends stopped calling me. Some told me I talked too much about my condition. I don't know how I would've dealt with this without my parents' support, as sometimes I was unable even to walk from my room to the kitchen, let alone stand and prepare a meal. I couldn't drive, so I relied on my dad to take me to numerous appointments. Shopping was extremely difficult.

Although using public transport was difficult while I was in a wheelchair, I continued going to the office and working full time. In spite of attending counselling and taking antidepressants and antipsychotics, my symptoms weren't improving. What's more, I got severe jaw clenching that made me unable to chew solid food, and my speech became slurred. The neuropsychiatrist gave me more medication, but it didn't help. I ended up as an inpatient at a neuropsychiatry service. My dystonia did improve there, but improvements and setbacks were happening even before my hospitalization, so the success is hard to attribute to hospitalization. While hospitalized, I attended CBT classes and physiotherapy, and participated in many of their other programmes.

Six months later, my dystonia worsened in the knee. I thought, considering how much work I put into counselling, surely my doctor will realize, there is something more to this than just psychological factors. But, to my disappointment, he told me I wasn't trying hard enough. I decided to leave him because he was giving me too much stress. I asked my GP to send a referral to a movement disorder clinic. A neurologist accepted me and told me I didn't need a psychiatrist. They couldn't really cure me, but at least they were not making things worse.

Two years ago, I stumbled on an article on women masking their autism and I realized that I am one of those women. Now I wonder if my autism could be a missing piece in this FND puzzle? In any case, it makes more sense to me than the theory of suppressed emotions.

Eleven years later, I'm still having dystonia, but it is not as intense as it was at the beginning. Now I am able to go for short walks using a cane [walking stick]. I've got used to other people's stares and I don't even pay attention to them anymore. I still feel tightness in my jaw, but I'm able to chew and speak clearly. Unfortunately, I've also had long Covid, so my energy is now even more limited. I never stopped working full time in accounting. Sometimes I work from home and sometimes in the office, depending on my health.

I have noticed that long Covid is very similar to FND in many aspects. In fact, now I'm a member of FND and long Covid support groups on Facebook, so I have posts from both groups on my timeline. Many times, I have to do a double take to see if the person complaining of the symptoms has FND or long Covid. Could this be because the virus causes changes in the brain's functionality? Could FND be related to the immune system dysfunction? Those things remain to be seen.

48

Learning With and From People with FND: A Neurologist's Story

Neurologist, 16 years' experience
of working with FND, UK

I had been training in neurology for a few months when an elderly woman using a wheelchair came in with a suspected stroke. She had diagnoses of Parkinson's disease and multiple sclerosis; both made about 25 years previously. She had been unable to walk since. She did not have a stroke, but I was intrigued by her husband telling me he saw her walk in the night six weeks earlier. I was surprised not to see signs of either Parkinson's or multiple sclerosis, but good strength in the chair, so I said: 'shall we try and walk?'. She started vomiting profusely, but once that settled, she gave it a try and was able to walk soon after. Within a few days, she was walking relatively normally and did not need a wheelchair. When she left hospital soon after, she believed the stroke had cured her. Her family struggled to understand how the diagnosis had been wrong and how they had helped her for so long when this was not needed anymore now. When I met her one year later she could still walk.

Now, more than 15 years later, I reflect on the risk of undiagnosis and that beliefs of how people improve might not always matter, but I am still excited to see how enabling people with FND to recognize the nature of their disorder and joining them on a therapeutic journey can be associated with dramatic improvements. Now, doing a weekly FND clinic and seeing many people with FND in my general neurology work, I learn something from every person. I share book recommendations, for different people and different symptoms, and last week I was very touched when a patient brought many copies of *It's All in Your Head* (O'Sullivan, 2021) (the title is not great) and *A Leg to Stand On* by Oliver Sacks (1984) for me to share with the doctors in training. He felt they should read more about FND, and he is right of course. We learn from stories.

I have heard people literally say that the penny dropped when they were shown Hoover's sign or how a severely tremulous spiral drawing normalized after tapping with the other hand. It is wonderful to see how these complex mechanisms of discrepancy between perceived involuntary and automatic movements become visible.

Over the years, I have learned how, when I try and support a therapeutic relationship, surprising things happen; from a lady with an eye that has been closed for years opening when she cries, to people who can't walk but can run (in the hospital wards). I have learned how to talk to people in the distressed state of a prolonged dissociative (functional) seizure and help them calm down. I have heard beautiful singing from people who struggled to speak, have a severe stutter, or foreign accent syndrome. I have heard normal swearing in someone who could hardly speak. I have seen constantly moving ears and toes being distracted and entrained.

Strange symptoms have started to make sense; someone with left-sided symptoms that included anaesthesia of the forearm around the area of a tattoo with the name of a beloved deceased relative developed autoscopy [where a person perceives the environment from a different perspective]; there were minutes when she would see herself from above. If your body or a body part does not feel as if it belongs to you, as many people with FND say, an out-of-body experience makes sense. When this is the case, it also makes sense for people to lose ticklishness, sometimes in one body part or all over, when they get FND symptoms, but also that it returns when they improve. When doing therapeutic sedation, dramatic changes can happen; during a relaxed conversation involving humour, suddenly there is a normalization of the prolonged fixed dystonia and the person regains the ability to feel and walk. Often it just gives people a nudge rather than being sufficient as a standalone treatment but nonetheless the hope of improvement is powerful.

I have also learned that what is visible (e.g., the paralysis or tremor) is not necessarily where treatment helps; sometimes helping with the workplace, benefits, migraine or PTSD has a much bigger impact, as can reducing medication. Over time, I have improved my engagement with families and friends, moving beyond the person affected in isolation. Importantly, people with FND have often been confused by the medical system; different professionals giving seemingly conflicting advice with insufficiently understood and explained incidental findings, from low copper to degenerative changes and pineal cysts. This makes it hard at times, when our narratives do not overlap enough for a therapeutic relationship. Such relationships can form over time, however, so when the door remains open, sometimes people return. I have learned to use the words of the patient as a window to understanding; for example, when people say they ignore or fight their body. I now write my letters to the patients so they feel at the centre, which is where they should be. I do not say 'we will fix it for you', but 'we will join you on your journey and guide and help you'. I hope I can join many more people on their FND journey in avoiding medical harm, understanding and improving their own and their loved one's lives; breaking intergenerational habits can be a good outcome in itself. People with FND have shown me how I can be a better doctor, something for which I am eternally grateful.

References

O'Sullivan, S. (2015). *It's All In Your Head*. London: Vintage.
Sacks, O. (1984). *A Leg to Stand On*. New York, NY: Summit Books.

A Poem: A Life Unmoored

Female, 56 years old, Canada

FUNCTIONAL MOVEMENT DISORDER

My way was so smooth,
As I danced to life's groove,
Now cast down 'n broken,
Can't ride with no tokens.
I wonder what I, can now signify,
A bird up on high,
A worm meant to die?
Can a soul accomplish if already diminished.
Toxic thoughts on the stream,
Of my thoughts and my dreams,
Burning they provide,
Flames that feast on my pride.
Have I courage of an ant,
Tiny yet bold with intent
To bend the world to his will,
Working, building seldom still
Small soldier you
Give me pause
Do I stumble just because,
My world reeks of ashes,
Seen through broken glasses.

Can I be whole yet in part,
Discover and birth a new art,
Formed from what I can see
Even partially,
That can be what I do,
Not comparing to you
If that I achieve
Then I'll no longer grieve.

50

Observations from a Front Row Seat

Dual trained neurologist-psychiatrist
and researcher, 14 years' experience
of working with FND, US

As a neurologist-psychiatrist engaged in the clinical care of patients with FND, I wanted to take this opportunity to share a few clinical insights that many of my institutional colleagues have heard me discuss – but on a topic that I have not yet spoken about in a public forum in any detail.

One of my favourite clinical experiences is meeting with a patient that has had a positive treatment response. In those follow-up visits, I ask them, 'What did you learn over the course of treatment?' and, 'What aspects of treatment did you find particularly helpful or unhelpful?' This is where I've had some of my most gratifying moments and insights as a clinician and researcher. In some instances, I've found that patients will share in detail their own 'personal equation' for developing FND. At times, they identify and report back on nuanced connections between thoughts, emotions, behaviours, life factors and functional neurological symptoms that were not apparent to them (and in many regards also not apparent to the clinical team) during the early stages of care. When I have a front row seat to witness this growth – including at times overt endorsements of how interconnected physical health and mental health are – it gives me chills. It is these moments that prove energizing, providing the motivation to persevere in the setting of other clinical, healthcare system and funding challenges. It is also these encounters that emphasize the importance of adding the voice of those who have recovered (or markedly improved) from FND to the range of important patient advocacy perspectives.

I'd like to offer a specific example. I remember a patient that I met with a few years ago, where I asked her, 'What did you learn over the course of treatment?' She referenced our initial clinical interview, where during the middle portions she remembered that I had asked her questions about anxiety – and she stated no to all those questions. She subsequently recounted that over the course of treatment, 'I learned that some of the thoughts and behaviours that I was using are what others might call anxiety' (quote paraphrased). I found this statement enlightening – in part because I remembered the initial interview where I observed that she was flushed in the face and seemingly had an anxious affect, while concurrently not endorsing negative emotions in the moment. This is an example of a clinical observation that has helped catalyse research questions.

51

A Psychologist's Personal Experience with Functional Seizures

Clinical psychologist living with FND, Australia

FUNCTIONAL SEIZURES

One day I woke up and I couldn't walk properly. It started with a hobble, and then over the next 48 hours, my gait progressed to a stagger and then I collapsed on my arrival at the hospital emergency department. I remember collapsing when I clambered out of the car. I remember being surrounded by emergency staff asking me to try to communicate or move my body. I could hear them, but I could neither speak nor move. The rest of that night in the emergency ward is hard to recall.

For the next two weeks, I lay in bed while doctors tried to figure out what to do with me. Months of scans, blood tests, a lumbar puncture and a week of epilepsy monitoring followed. Test after test showed that I had a healthy brain. But there was something wrong because I experienced daily episodes of dissociation that caused my body to become limp. I lay in bed, unable to move my body or communicate through a wall of mental fog and slurred speech. Walking was a tremendous and exhausting effort. I had numerous falls, and I would collapse when sitting. I couldn't sleep at night because of inexplicable chronic pain in my lower back. The less I slept, the worse my symptoms became. The most debilitating aspects of my new FND life were the daily episodes of NES that would last up to an hour at a time.

I had been a psychologist for 19 years. I had a thriving private practice, and I was fit and healthy. When I came out of the hospital, I was lost. I had a diagnosis but no direction. Over the next six months, I read as much as possible about FND, and, over time, I put together a team of health professionals from all over the country to help me rebuild my life.

FND is one of the earliest psychological conditions known. Hippocrates called it the 'wandering womb'; Freud called it 'conversion disorder'. From what we know now, FND is not just a psychological disorder, but a complex neurological condition with a myriad of biological, contextual, and psychological factors. The world's leading experts are working hard to develop gold standard treatments for FND. The condition is nebulous, complex, and variable from person to person in its severity and its symptom profile. For those living with FND, our experiences are similar, but our stories are very different.

I would not be where I am without the dedication of my yoga therapist, occupational therapist, neuropsychologist, clinical psychologist, psychiatrist, neurologist, acupuncturist, dietitian and physiotherapist. I am eternally grateful to my neuropsychologist, who introduced me to virtual reality gaming. I found that apps hijacked my gait disorder, pulled me out of the prodrome of dissociative attacks, and curtailed the agony of my chronic pain. Yoga therapy helped me to walk again. Occupational therapy gave me the tools to conserve my energy to prevent symptom flare-ups, function in everyday life and rebuild my career.

I have come a long way since the onset of my symptoms. I live with FND, but FND is no longer my life. I have learned much about the condition through many hours of conversation, study and treatment. I hope that the tools that have helped me get to where I am are tools that I can share to help others with FND.

52

Processing Traumatic Events

Psychotherapist, nine years' experience
of working with FND, UK

Sarah [pseudonym] was in her thirties, single and had no children. She was referred to our neuropsychology team to help manage her non-epileptic episodes (functional seizures). She had a diagnosis of NEAD as well as epilepsy. She presented with frequent twitching in her left leg and her vision was sometimes blurred. She also had twitching in her left eye.

Sarah was frustrated; it took a long time for her FND diagnosis to be confirmed. At the first appointment, she was angry and fed up. She did not want yet another diagnosis. The complexity of FND often leads to misdiagnosis. There is frequent use of unnecessary clinical procedures. Sarah presented many times to A&E with suspected uncontrolled epilepsy. She was investigated for cardiological problems and possible strokes. She felt she had been overly cared for and then dismissed many times. She had felt scared and then been told to go home. She felt very confused.

On her first session, she had already seen many doctors, nurses and two psychologists, whom she reported she had not got on well with. Taking the risk to sit with her NEAD episodes was high; however, her epilepsy was thought to be under control. In the first appointment, she was quiet, angry and withdrawn. She sat close to the door, wanting a quick exit. She reported that life had been unkind and unfair and she told me she had been dealt a bad hand.

I guess it must feel like that to patients with FND. She said, 'I must have been a bitch in my previous life.' The world of FND *is* unfair. She struggled with sensory overload. The light hurt her eyes and she had difficulty concentrating, which impacted her work and her finances. She was tired. She sat with her head in her hands and asked me, 'Why am I getting these symptoms, why me?' All I could say was, 'We don't know, but I guess we can try and work it out together.'

I continued to see Sarah in clinic every fortnight. After 16 sessions, she disclosed that she had been raped. She was recovering from an epileptic attack when she was raped. She was vulnerable and had no control to stop it or to shout for help. She was sexually assaulted multiple times. This had never been disclosed, never been reported until now.

During the course of two years, I supported her to engage and build trust in relationships, and helped her recognize when she was emotionally disconnecting and needed to reconnect. We worked on stabilization, using grounding strategies and the traffic light system. She learned to recognize when she was in the threat system, when her pressure cooker was building. Managing stress, emotional build-up and challenging thoughts all contributed to stabilization. She learned to assert herself.

Before accepting her diagnosis, Sarah wanted a second opinion. I felt this alone was a therapeutic intervention. She was asking for her needs to be met and was willing to go to a medical appointment. So, I agreed to support her with this. After this second opinion, we worked on acceptance and education of FND. We built a good relationship. We worked on her trauma, helping to process the trauma events.

Sarah and I noticed her symptoms evolving. They reduced, and her quality of life improved. Over the two years, we continued to check in on weekly triggers, sometimes normalizing these. Week by week, she moved forward – to the first committed relationship and teething difficulties a relationship brings, then the purchase of her first house. These situations are anxiety provoking to many but in recognizing normal anxious situations from life-threatening ones, Sarah became grounded. She became stabilized and began to trust others.

I doubt this could have been done without the support of psychotherapy. Over time, she learned to control her NEAD; her twitches would come and go. The episodes were often triggered when she felt in a difficult and 'trapped' situation. She managed hospital appointments and improved her quality of life overall. I know psychotherapy helped her, with a combination of methods such as acceptance commitment therapy, CBT, EMDR, and psychodynamic interpersonal therapy. We used education from the polyvagal therapy, explaining FND. Sarah learned to listen to her body and recognize early warning signs.

Sarah's therapy faded out. We had bigger gaps between sessions as she started to gain control. The two years felt like a rollercoaster, but it was just the time she needed to heal. We finally said goodbye.

I often think of Sarah when patients are triggered with similar presentations, when they are angry and disconnected. It wasn't easy with Sarah, but she gives me hope. Sarah became a mum and when I received a card with the picture of her beautiful baby, the message read, 'We welcomed our baby into the world.'

53

Raising Awareness about Functional Seizures

FUNCTIONAL SEIZURES

Female, 29 years old, UK

I have a dual diagnosis of epilepsy and NEAD (functional seizures).
After many years of my seizures being uncontrolled and medications being stockpiled within my system and not working, I was given a diagnosis of NEAD. When I was first given the diagnosis, I did not understand what it was. I had never heard of it and was given limited information when spoken to by a doctor. So, when researching it myself, I interpreted the information negatively. This negativity was then further reinforced by negative comments from a health professional who was treating me. I did not want another label, let alone one nobody understood, but having hospital admissions on a regular basis and visits to A&E and doctors telling you and your family that you're taking a bed somebody else needs because these seizures are not real, it just further reinforces that negativity you already have around the diagnosis.

The thing is, I had not ended up in A&E because of NEAD. I had been taken by the paramedics because I had a seizure and had injuries from it. NEAD episodes just followed this. And this was the treatment I received. Follow-up appointments with my neurologist just focused on my epilepsy, because I was told NEAD is not treated by medication. I was on a waiting list for the NEAD service. My family and I felt as if we were alone and left to navigate our way through this diagnosis.

My family has been great and really adapted well to it and taken on the knowledge that we have either found ourselves or eventually been given. This is happening, let's deal with it. Me on the other hand, I have been closed off from it and, to an extent, in denial. I do not want this to happen and if I ignore it, maybe it will go away. Unfortunately, it has not. I eventually got seen by the NEAD service, but it did not last long. I initially had a group session only to be told I was not allowed to join in these sessions as I had a dual diagnosis. I then began having one-to-one sessions in which, yet again, the professional I came in contact with did not know how to communicate with people, especially those with NEAD, which is ironic considering it was an NEAD service.

I felt uncomfortable and invalidated by the comments being made so I personally made the choice to leave the service. However, I was re-referred about 18 months later when both my seizures and NEAD episodes became severely uncontrolled, and I had to spend six weeks in hospital because of them. My feelings and beliefs around the diagnosis already made me reluctant to go to any appointments but my past experiences were making it even harder. But what did I have to lose, as at this point I was not living a life? I was spending more time in hospital than I was out, because I was so uncontrolled. The professional I saw this time was different; there were no negative comments, there was no pushing any beliefs on to me and no telling me I was there because I had fake seizures. I still found it difficult, but there was something telling me to give it a go this time.

I have a better understanding of what NEAD is as a whole now, but I still have negative feelings towards having the diagnosis. This is something I am aware of, and I know I need to work on. I do believe it is because of the treatment and comments I experienced when I first received the diagnosis. The positive thing is that having that understanding does not make me view NEAD negatively. I know this for certain because I have been lucky enough to not only be diagnosed with it but encounter someone else who has been diagnosed with it within my workplace. The people I worked with did not know what it was, had not heard of it and made similar comments to this person to what I received when I was experiencing episodes. I explained to them in detail what NEAD was and how their comments could be damaging. I explained that not having knowledge about something like this can bring fear and anxiety and that is probably where the comments were coming from, but those comments, if heard by the person having the episode, would remain with them forever and could become their own beliefs. I also spoke with the individual experiencing NEAD; it was a new diagnosis and they did not know much about it. We had a conversation about NEAD and how it is okay to have it.

In that situation, I was so positive about NEAD, yet I still hold negativity around my own diagnosis. I resent having it and feel like a fraud for having 'fake seizures'. There's nothing actually wrong with me, is there? This has been an internal battle that has been going on for years now. I am working on it with the help of a professional I see at the NEAD service, and I am grateful for the hard work, patience and passion they have for the job and for me. They have helped me view both professionals and NEAD in a different way. I only wish the process of getting a diagnosis was a lot smoother and professional across the board, not limited to specialized professionals who have a lot more knowledge around NEAD and can prevent people experiencing this negativity because of lack of knowledge and fear.

Author's mother

From the age of 11, my daughter was diagnosed with photosensitive epilepsy, which we have struggled with for many years as it was not controlled. We then found out after many weeks in hospital that she suffered from NEAD, which we knew nothing about. At this point, very limited information was given to us and we were just told we would be given a follow-up appointment with the NEAD service which would help explain everything. The wait to be seen in this service was long and in the meantime, her seizures and NEAD episodes were happening daily, so as a family we had to learn about it ourselves.

My daughter continued being admitted to hospital where we experienced negative feedback in both A&E and on the wards. At one point, when I went to visit her when she had been admitted as an inpatient, another patient informed me that they had been looking after her because the nurses had not come, even though other patients had pressed their buzzer to tell them she was having a seizure. When I complained about this, I was told by a nurse that my daughter was faking the seizure, and that was why they had left her, as they had patients who were really poorly to look after. During an NEAD episode, my husband was also asked to take her home by a doctor, as the hospital did not understand the diagnosis.

Another negative experience was when I got a call asking me to go to A&E because my daughter was in hospital. When I got there, a nurse had told me she had had several seizures and they were taking her down for a scan. While waiting for the scan, my daughter continued to have what they thought were seizures, and because they lasted longer than five minutes, she was given rescue medication. I asked the doctor if she really needed this as these were NEAD episodes/seizures but I was dismissed and ignored, and so was the information I was providing. It was only when the doctor swapped shifts and another doctor took over and spoke to me after witnessing an NEAD episode that I was listened to and that the medication that was being given to her each time was stopped.

The doctor asked how I knew they were different from her tonic-clonic (epileptic) seizures and explained he had heard about NEAD but had limited knowledge in this area so he would be taking guidance from me if that was okay. He was willing to learn about the area and took notes to look back on. He asked for the nurses to call every time a seizure or episode happened so he could see them and learn. He also took time to speak to my daughter as a person and not a condition. After several hours, the seizures stopped. Because he was calm and positive towards the situation, this helped both my daughter and me. His enthusiasm to learn about NEAD did not go unnoticed and was appreciated. However, it should not require experiences like this for a doctor to learn. There should be more awareness of NEAD so there is less negativity around it from both healthcare professionals and people you meet every day.

54

Bird in the Cage

Mental health occupational therapist, seven years'
experience of working with FND, Australia

She came to the session with her husband and by the end of the 90 minutes, her life had begun to take a different turn. She spoke about a shaking tremor and NES. He spoke about her nightmares and poor sleep. The family stressors were huge as they had a child with a serious illness. Just before leaving the session, I always ask, is there anything else you would like to add. This question hit the jackpot, 'Yes, I would just like to say my marriage is dysfunctional and needs help.' Bullseye. This is what we worked on for the next two years.

She discovered she was in an abusive controlling relationship. 'He didn't hit me', this factor confused her, and she believed for many years that things weren't so bad. Her baseline for healthy relationships was low. But slowly she began to put up boundaries within the relationship, saying 'no', talking about things that were never said, and slowly her FND symptoms began to lessen.

Then one day, she left her cage with her little baby birds and found a house to live in. He found her as he had a tracker on her phone, but she installed cameras and told him to go. She will eventually fly away but right now, she sits on the outside of the cage as she needs to process, remember and feel. She has stopped having nightmares, she sleeps well and her children sleep well too.

Her headaches are infrequent and her shaking has stopped; she has a new look and feels great.

This story is typical of the women who come to sessions because they have FND and a back story of being too nice (can't say no), too accommodating (nothing is too much trouble), too helpful (I can do that for you), too useful in the workplace (literally doing everything from sales to accounting to training and generally not being paid for it). In my experience, those women generally have one-sided weakness resembling stroke and sometimes shakes and tremors. They have been working very hard, keeping households together, workplaces organized and usually caring for older parents. They are exhausted but keep pushing on because they always have, and others expect it of them.

I have also observed that other women with dissociative (functional) attacks have been, or are currently, in abusive, violent relationships with partners or husbands. These men not only abuse them but also often leave these women with no access to money or with very limited access. These women have no idea how much money they have as a couple. Some women are actually given pocket money by their husband, such as a mere $20 a week to buy any necessities, including sanitary products. They have mostly been abused and/or neglected as children, either by their father or their mother's boyfriend, or their grandfather. They mostly go on to choose men who control and abuse them and then they go on to develop symptoms of FND. This is my typical caseload – all in a day's work at the hospital public outpatient department.

I am trauma trained and can recognize narcissism because I realized way back, I would need this skill to actually be able to help these women. I have seen countless women come through the service and they keep coming. The phrase I hear most is, 'I have never told anyone this before' and I just say, 'It's okay, this is a safe space and I'm here to listen.' I wish I could say I am shocked and surprised, but nothing surprises me now. That said, I'm not burnt out. But I am passionate about this mission to free all the caged birds. It's my job to just sit in my room day after day, helping women to unlock the cage door and eventually fly away. It gives me great delight to hear women come back and say, 'You would be proud of me, I said this or I did this.' I am someone in their life who cares about them and who stays for the long haul.

We start with the basics: sleep, food and moving the body. Teaching deep breathing and how to listen to the body using body scans, grounding or tapping helps some. I'm an eclectic practitioner, as one size never fits all. Mostly, I teach them that they are worthy, and they matter. Most of this work is very private; these are private matters and so will never reach the research forum, as when they fly, they fly. I can say I have assisted many hundreds of broken birds to leave the cage and fly. That is an honour and a privilege. What I would like to see moving forward is more public outpatient, long-term assistance for women with FND, socio-economic and gender equality – not much really, but a vision to work towards.

55

Challenges in the Healthcare System

Psychologist, six years' experience of
working with FND, Argentina

My work with Analía [pseudonym] began two years ago and
despite improvements in her affective and dissociative symptoms
and in her quality of life, we still continue to address and discuss psychoeducational issues. Analía is a patient who must be
reminded that consulting with many professionals brings confusion. It seems that for her, it is like not giving in to the disease.
She perceives that this keeps her active in the fight. I perceive
that she has a hard time accepting that the work to be done involves
her thoughts, emotions, coping styles, and even connecting with
past events.

What I read when I had just started my journey as a therapist
for patients with functional symptoms becomes real: for many
patients, explaining that their condition has a psychological and
not a structural origin is not reassuring. I wonder, does it have to
be the other way around? Does the fact that Analía's seizures and
movements do not have a structural origin have to reassure her? I
remember a phrase that she said me when we started: 'If this is
because of my head I'm done for; my head is very hard to change.'
Working with Analía, as with all patients with dissociative seizures,
has involved moments of great achievements and moments of

setbacks, and sustaining frustration in moments of setbacks or stagnation is difficult for both the patient and the professional. She no longer has dissociative (functional) seizures today; she has been able to control them with grounding exercises, mainly using her sense of smell (with a perfume) and hearing (her daughter's voice reminding her not to 'leave').

Currently, the main problem is her functional movement. Analía presents with tremors in her legs, which, in the most serious moments, turn into spasms. At times, she has no control of her left arm and her voice trembles. She is in a wheelchair because she cannot walk. Her movements have decreased in intensity, but they are the main obstacle for Analía, stopping her from being able to live independently. Her current life contrasts with her past life: an athlete, a worker, a spouse and a carer, without help, of her daughter. Treatment recommendations suggest that patients should lead an active life, carrying out activities that do not pose a danger to them. They recommend that patients should continue their work activities and, as far as functional movements are concerned, complement mental health treatments with physiotherapy and rehabilitation.

Meeting these objectives in this country is difficult. Analía is a privileged person when it comes to health coverage here, since she has one of the best prepaid plans. Even so, she is a victim of the lack of knowledge of professionals about these disorders and the mismanagement of healthcare. For example, she has not yet been able to start her physical rehabilitation. Although today we are in the final stretch of achieving it, Analía has had to request endless consultations with her prepaid professionals, who insisted that her diagnosis was epilepsy. On the other hand, the clinicians in the rehabilitation centres argued that her problem was not physical but psychiatric and, for that reason, she could not undergo physical therapy. In addition, Analía has been without a therapeutic companion for a year and a half due to lack of response from her health insurance. In Argentina, a therapeutic companion ('acompañante terapéutico') works as a member of a therapeutic team. In the case of Analía, the objective is to accompany her in her daily life to achieve certain therapeutic objectives, such as achieving her independence in certain tasks, going out on social occasions, among others. For this reason, she spends her days locked up in her house, since she cannot move on her own. Despite having the cognitive abilities to continue working, her institution denies her this possibility. Situations like these are extremely frustrating for patients, but also for the professionals. As a professional, I feel my hands are tied in the face of a health system that does not understand and does not include this type of disorder. So, I ask myself, how is a patient with FND going to accept their condition, when not even the health system, which should help them, recognizes it?

I also work in a public hospital and there the problems that need attention become more acute. A collapsed health system, with a lack of knowledge in FND, patients with few economic resources, with complicated social situations. I think that if one does not live in Argentina, one cannot imagine these difficulties. I belong to a group of professionals who investigate and treat patients with functional disorders. I believe that our main commitment is to be able to transmit our knowledge to as many health professionals as possible. In this way, we can best help patients and professionals.

56

Light at the End of the Tunnel

Female, 33 years old, UK

FUNCTIONAL COGNITIVE AND
MOVEMENT DISORDER

It all started suddenly and for absolutely no reason at all. At first, I had pins and needles and weakness in my right arm and was referred to rheumatology. They initially thought that I had a slipped disc in my neck or had done something to my shoulder. After several scans, I was diagnosed with a Chiari malformation type I (where the brain pushes on the spinal canal), and was referred to neurology. Two years passed with very little interventional help and, having been told that my Chiari malformation was not the cause of my issues, I was almost losing hope.

I asked for a second opinion and was told that I had FND. This, however, was a 'suspected' cause of all the other symptoms that I had developed. Having done a little bit of research and coming across an article at my local hospital (where I work), I contacted the neurologist directly and asked how I could get a referral to her. Within two weeks, I had an appointment and an official diagnosis, with proper support and advice regarding what to do if things were to worsen. I was also sent to the neurophysiologist and a neuropsychologist.

The neurophysiologist was absolutely brilliant. After an hour and a half with her, she explained exactly where my triggers had come from and how to overcome them going forward. She spent 20-30 minutes talking to my mum, asking her similar questions without me in the room, which was completely fine, but it was so my mum could be open and honest with her.

I have since left my job and joined a different department where I have been supported a lot more, and occupational health has also been a massive help. I have good days and bad days but at least I know my triggers. I have fewer bad days where I completely seize up and can't move out of bed. I also have fewer occurrences of chronic fatigue knocking me out for a week, and I'm better able to find ways to concentrate on larger tasks. At one point, FND completely consumed me, and I was not me anymore. My whole identity revolved around my symptoms and pain levels. Although it is difficult, there is light at the end of the tunnel. Mentally, I had to tell myself that I was more than I was giving myself credit for. As soon as I stopped believing that FND was going to ruin and control my life, things turned around for the better. Although FND is predominantly physical, in the sense of signs and symptoms, I do believe that a large part of it is mental, in the sense that people can become blindsided by the label of FND.

57

The Unpredictability of FND

Female, 37 years old, New Zealand

FUNCTIONAL MOVEMENT DISORDER

A brief peek into my FND journey: I have had a history of health quirks. Hypermobility syndrome, irritable bowel syndrome and possible celiac disease. I did have an eating disorder in my teens but feel that is another world away. Two years ago, we were due to fly home after a five-month trip visiting my husband's family in another country. Covid-19 changed everything and I never got to go home; and I wonder if the grief of not knowing when or if I'll see loved ones again is part of why I am here now.

Funnily enough, I was feeling in the best place mentally when it all kicked off. We had a house, great church family and a gorgeous puppy. After a week of being convinced I must be having blood sugar issues – sudden intense bouts of hunger and shakes that would take me to bed and keep me there for ages – I went out to a Bible study session. After answering a phone call – standing, walking away and back again – my shakes returned. But this time, they weren't leaving. My right leg got worse and worse. My friend drove me to the hospital. Hours later, I was discharged with some medication but no answers. After another two trips to A&E, I was admitted to hospital for two nights. I had many violent episodes of 'tremors' (the word never seems enough somehow when it leaves your heart soaring and your body caked in sweat and aches). I did have an MRI scan of my brain, which was all clear. I got sent home, awash with brain-muddling medicine and a referral to psychiatry, with the words 'the mind is a powerful thing' echoing, not so comfortingly, in my ears.

I couldn't walk. My friend had to find a wheelchair to get me to the car. Some days later I called my GP's office to ask what to do about the fact I couldn't walk, as it kept setting off episodes. I got a physiotherapy visit a week or so later, and she brought me a cane – a small, crook-handled blessing. I had tremors pretty much consistently for a long time, along with brain fog, incredible fatigue, myoclonic jerks, a strange new walk. My propensity for violent 'tremor' episodes would upset those around me. One time, at church, I was triggered by some loud noises, and I ended up trying to comfort those who were around me while half my body did its thing.

I only got my official diagnosis very recently. I had relied on the fact that on one of my A&E discharge notes, it mentioned 'possible conversion disorder', so, I had researched it. I found the new, up-to-date terms and definitions. I became well acquainted with https://neurosymptoms.org and learned to accept the ups and downs and to look for ways to try and overcome it. I have just had a good week during which I was able to walk the dog frequently, albeit with a not-perfect gait, but without constantly needing to use a stick. Two days ago, I had another episode. This time, the effects have remained. My walking has deteriorated a lot, and I am full of tremors and weakness and peculiar brain feelings again. But it's okay, because I understand more. I will keep trying to learn, and to share with others. It's how we can best deal with this thing – this fascinating, frustrating, fluctuating creature we call FND.

Postscript

Some months after writing this, I went from having my worst day to going into approximately 95 per cent remission, and have continued until the present day. I am enjoying life, even being active at the gym again multiple times a week. I try to remember to really appreciate my physical ability, knowing how unpredictable FND can be, and how many suffer for so long. I still have some symptoms, but nothing major or debilitating – mostly visual/fatigue.

58

Functional Seizures in Adults with an Intellectual (Learning) Disability

Clinical psychologist and researcher, eight years' experience of working with FND, UK

I was part way through my training to become a clinical psychologist on placement at a health service for adults with intellectual disabilities (also known as learning disabilities). Sitting in the weekly referrals meeting, we were discussing individuals who had been referred to psychology for treatment as they were experiencing difficulties with their mental health. Among the clients who were discussed, the service lead explained we may be receiving a referral soon for someone who was experiencing functional seizures. He then turned to me saying that we were in a good position to support the person given my previous experience of working with this clinical group. Over the previous six years or so, I had been involved in a number of research projects, including completing my doctorate on the condition. Sitting in the meeting, however, I felt a sense of embarrassment, as, until that point, I had barely given any thought to the condition in the context of people with intellectual disabilities. I smiled in response just hoping I wouldn't be asked any questions. After the meeting had finished, I was left with a feeling of dread at the thought that I may be asked to help this person very soon, and I had more questions than I did answers. The client was not referred to our service in the end, and although I cannot remember the reason why or much about the client, that feeling of inadequacy has stayed with me.

● ● ●

An intellectual disability is a lifelong condition that is present before adulthood (18 years of age). Some individuals are diagnosed while they are still a child or adolescent and receive appropriate support and care; however, others may not receive a diagnosis until later in life. An intellectual disability is characterized by significant difficulties in:

- intellectual functioning, meaning the person may experience challenges when learning new skills, understanding information, remembering things, communicating, reading, writing, managing their emotions and in social situations. On standardized measures of IQ, the person would score significantly below the average of the general population
- social or adaptive functioning, and so individuals may need support with everyday activities that could range from personal care, chores around the house, engaging in their communities and living independently.

An intellectual disability differs from a learning difficulty, such as dyslexia or dyspraxia. A learning difficulty means an individual will have a problem with a specific task, whereas an intellectual disability is a global difficulty, causing the individual to experience problems across a range of daily activities. People can be classified as having mild, moderate, severe, or profound intellectual disabilities, which reflect the level of difficulties and support they may need. An intellectual disability cannot be cured, but individuals can [should] be supported to live a fulfilling and happy life.

● ● ●

People with an intellectual disability are at a greater risk of experiencing inequalities in everyday life, even in healthcare. For example, I have read countless studies on functional seizures where individuals with intellectual disabilities are underrepresented, where they have been excluded from the study without a reason being provided or a discussion of what measures the authors had taken to support this group to engage. Even in my own research into FND, I recognize that we did not adapt aspects of the study with this population in mind. It is probably such practices that have contributed – in part – to my lack of awareness of the condition in this population.

For many years, it was believed that people with an intellectual disability did not have the cognitive functioning to suffer from mental health difficulties or benefit from psychological treatments. Fortunately, we have moved on from such ideas and there is an ever-growing evidence base demonstrating the positive outcomes associated with psychological interventions when tailored to the individual's needs, ability and circumstance. And in fact, we now know that rates of mental health problems in this population are greater than those in the general population. This appears to also include functional seizures, with research suggesting that approximately 10 per cent (and in some cases up to 45 per cent) of patient groups with functional seizures also have an intellectual disability. This figure is greater than estimates of the prevalence of intellectual disabilities in the general population, which stand at about 1 per cent.

As in those with functional seizures and without an intellectual disability, the true prevalence may be higher, with this group likely (or possibly more likely) to experience common barriers to gaining a diagnosis and treatment as often described by others with functional seizures. For example, epilepsy and repetitive motor behaviours are more prevalent in people with intellectual disabilities, which may pose additional challenges when making a differential diagnosis – particularly for those who struggle to communicate their experiences to others.

Diagnostic overshadowing is also a concern, which is when the psychosocial difficulties an individual experiences are assumed to just be a manifestation of their intellectual disability, as opposed to a mental health condition such as functional seizures. There is also the argument that the condition is even more of an 'orphan disorder', which does not have a clear home in traditional Western healthcare services. This may help to explain why people with functional seizures received multiple referrals to different specialities before receiving the correct diagnosis, and even then, there may not be a clear pathway for their treatment. Healthcare professionals working in mainstream services for functional seizures may believe those in intellectual disability specific services should be responsible for providing care for this group because of their specialist training in intellectual disabilities, and vice versa, those in intellectual disability services may feel they do not have the expertise to treat functional seizures. For example, I am now a qualified clinical psychologist working in the same health service for adults with an intellectual disability as discussed previously, and it is rare when someone from this sub-group is referred to us. I assume they are being supported by mainstream services for functional seizures, not receiving care, or their functional seizures have been misdiagnosed – which may be more common in those with intellectual disabilities than the general population.

● ● ●

When I consulted the literature to better understand the cause of functional seizures in people with intellectual disabilities, I noticed there was a tendency to interpret the seizures through a behavioural lens. In other words, seizures have been described as a response to what is happening in the individual's immediate environment and can be a way of communicating their (unmet) needs. Some authors have discussed the higher prevalence of epilepsy in this group and how family, friends and carers tend to respond to epileptic seizures, suggesting a functional seizure is positively reinforced by others due to increased attention and care, and therefore, is a learned behavioural response. This may present a lack of a nuanced understanding regarding cognitive, psychological and emotional processes which could help us to understand functional seizures in people with intellectual disabilities. Indeed, this notion is reflected in commonly described treatments that have been published, which tend to be more focused on behavioural modification and environmental adjustments. While psychological interventions, such as CBT, are the treatment of choice for functional seizures in the general population, it appears treatments for the condition in those with an intellectual disability are informed by approaches focusing more on behaviours than cognitions; that is, using a little c(ognitive) and big B(ehavioural) approach.

A recent review of functional seizures (also known as PNES) and intellectual disabilities postulates:

> ...it seems best to assume that there is little difference in the aetiology or function of PNES between those with and without ID, and that for most, PNES in ID are an involuntary mechanism which functions as a means of protecting the individual from a stimulus that is experienced as overwhelming, threatening or intolerable (Rawlings *et al.*, 2021)

In line with this notion, treatments for this group should explore and formulate the client's emotional and cognitive distress (in addition to behavioural and environmental factors) that may be triggering their functional seizures. Clients should be provided with the support, care and compassion that all individuals with the condition deserve and which, no doubt, play a crucial role in recovery.

I hope to have provided a brief overview of some salient themes on functional seizures in those with intellectual disabilities, which will contribute to the growing number of conversations about functional seizures more generally, and about their presentation in those from underrepresented groups more specifically, including those with additional needs. It was my fear that this book would be another platform where their experiences would sadly not be reflected. Perhaps if I had read a similar chapter as this several years ago, I would have had a greater awareness when that individual was discussed in the referrals meeting during my training. By failing to research functional seizures in those with intellectual disabilities, there is a real risk of unintentionally contributing to the inequalities in care and lower quality of life that is typically observed in this group.

Reference

Rawlings, G.H., Novakova, B., Beail, N. & Reuber, M. (2021). What do we know about non-epileptic seizures in adults with intellectual disability: A narrative review. *Seizure* 91, 437–446. https://doi.org/10.1016/j.seizure.2021.07.021

59

Heard: Recovering from Childhood Trauma

HEADACHES, BLACKOUTS, DISSOCIATIVE (FUNCTIONAL) SEIZURES, FUNCTIONAL STROKES, NUMBNESS

My diagnosis

Four years ago, I was rushed into hospital suffering from over 20 seizures and signs of a stroke. I stayed in hospital for over a week. Having had numerous scans, blood tests and a lumbar puncture, I lay in that bed, with no feeling from the neck down, slurred speech and nothing but tears in my eyes, trying to understand what on earth was going on! As soon as I was able to hobble to the toilet, I was discharged. Without any clear answers, I went to my GP. He asked me about my hospital admission and made a referral to neurology. I attended an appointment with a consultant. I had about three attacks while there. I was asked a number of questions and I hardly answered any of them honestly. The main question, I avoided completely. I was diagnosed with NEAD, also known as dissociative (functional) seizures, which translated to me as, 'What the flip!?!' I was put on the waiting list for neuropsychology. I just waited, wondering what I was going to say...

After a few regular visits to my GP, I was asked that question. Did I ever suffer any kind of trauma as a child? I felt my gut pull hard from the inside. I knew I couldn't lie; my body wouldn't let me. I instantly got really angry; what is it with these people and this question? But, for the first time in my life, I couldn't hold it in any longer, and I didn't want to either. From that point on, my GP took the lead and arranged all the medical assessments needed. Finally, I was being heard. I was referred to an outpatient department. There I was assessed and diagnosed with complex PTSD. So that was that, in my mind I was half-lunatic and half-freak. Lucky me! Another referral was made to psychology. Some days I struggled; it was the hardest first steps towards self-love I have ever walked. No regrets though, the knowledge and understanding I gained through both diagnoses was amazing!

The tough part

The police investigation was the hardest part. Laying everything out there. But there I was, freeing myself from my trauma. The investigating officers were kind and compassionate. And even though we never made it to court, it didn't seem to make that much difference. I was being heard. My abuser was now the scared and ashamed one. I was finally healing my hurt. I was finding my power.

Healing

And then it came. That dreaded appointment. Before attending my first appointment and even though I was relieved to have a diagnosis, part of me was still wondering whether I needed to go back for another assessment. But this was different, I was now under a neuropsychologist. It was here that I was helped to understand how my body responds to my triggers, including the physical symptoms. Counselling gave me a sense of freedom. I had finally found my safe space. I had a feeling of being offered lots of support by professionals, and it felt great, being so supported to overcome something I thought would destroy me. Was this what I needed? Was this the missing piece of the puzzle? It takes some time to really get your head around. And even with the understanding, care and compassion of some professionals, they cannot cure your symptoms. You have to learn to manage those symptoms on your own. As I was soon to learn...

Triggers

Handling my triggers is the hardest part of my recovery. I have since experienced more trauma. I was completely caught off guard with how my body reacted to being triggered. For the first time in my life, I am experiencing trauma and being fully aware of it, as well as my body's response to it. It can be both confusing and relieving at times. You may now wonder if all those appointments were worth it. To be honest, yes. My body is still healing. I am still a work in progress. Recovering from childhood trauma is not a quick fix.

The future

I am still trying to work through my past and present trauma. This time I am choosing not to numb the feelings with drugs and alcohol, like I did in my teenage years. I am still under neuropsychology and will soon be having EMDR. I am still learning to embrace my diagnosis in order to heal, and my only wish is that it is further understood by others, so people like me can gain the support we need, not just from the professionals involved in our care but from the wider community also. It's time we are all heard!

60

Walking the Dog

Male, 52 years old, UK

FUNCTIONAL SEIZURES

Just walking the dog... Dappled sunlight there was... Aroma of freshly cut grass with a gentle breeze, anticipation of time well spent and freedom with those I love. And then...simply nothing. A story I can't tell, as there are no memories... And so...here I am... emerging from this 'conscious coma' of dissociation. They say I walked... I talked... I shook... Did I? The evidence is only one of injury and pictorial horror where for some reason I have gone away, to a place even I can't record and am not privy to... Just away.

They ask, how do you feel...? Just fine I say, just a little fit. Get well soon chimes insistently...a constant peel of bells in the ear of a deaf man. Well from what? Where is this foreign land I used to call home?

I'm not though... My heart beats as a thousand drums... I breathe faster... Churning anxiety... Darkness... Who and what am I? Frightened, perplexed, sorrowful of what I have become... guilty for a sin I can't remember committing. Broken I suppose, as is the face that I once looked out of...

Future uncertain... Liberties of life restricted... A life now full of 'what ifs'. This is the reality.

Perhaps then... Without a story to tell... I wasn't there afterall; is to ask the self why...and indeed why now... I was just walking the dog. Such questions pose an 'easy' self-healing medicinal narrative that they say will better my understanding of the unfathomable. With absolute candour. My jury is out.

But...I have learned one thing. The fragility of life's apparent constant must never be taken for granted. Tomorrow will never be the same. Perhaps now is the time to forge a new and refreshed narrative for my life, one, in retrospect, I should have embraced earlier...

And so, my journey now starts... As to its end, only Father Time in his wisdom will guide me to my final resting place and destination. In the interim...I'll just keep walking the dog.

61

The Multidisciplinary Team: A Speech and Language Therapist's Perspective

Speech and language therapist, three years'
experience of working with FND, UK

My first experience of FND and working with this condition was less than one year into being a qualified speech and language therapist. I received a referral for a patient with communication difficulties who was based on a ward which usually specialized in tumours. I attended the ward, expecting to complete an initial communication assessment and likely provide advice and further input for dysarthria and dysphasia. However, during the assessment the profile was variable, unusual and unlike anything I had seen before: no comprehension deficit, written expressive language intact, inconsistent dysfluency, abnormal/tense breathing pattern and very tense facial muscles/jaw clamping. A nurse also explained to me that the patient could not open her mouth to eat and drink, which appeared in keeping with the patient's tense facial muscles and jaw clamping but again, my experience was neurology-based, therefore this presentation initially seemed confusing to me.

I discussed the case with colleagues, who queried if this patient may have FND. This was the first time I had heard of the condition. FND had not been covered within university teaching and it had not come up in any practical placements. At the time, none of the documented clinical notes for this patient across the multidisciplinary team made reference to the condition. After discussing the case with a colleague, I researched FND and we completed joint sessions while I built on my experience and confidence in this clinical area.

Our initial input centred around encouraging full multidisciplinary teamwork. Once neuropsychology explained the FND diagnosis to the patient, the plan from speech and language focused on education of how we articulate and produce voice and the functions of swallow and communication. We then began therapy with a variety of relaxation techniques to help ease the tension of facial muscles and jaw clamping, which jointly targeted improving her speech and the oral stage of dysphagia. One unexpected success was using desensitization methods alongside relaxation to help with the jaw clamping, which was quite severe in nature. The patient was only able to take fluids and soups via a straw for multiple weeks as she could not open her mouth wide enough to put food in with a spoon or fork. This led to significant pressure to support rehabilitation of the dysphagia symptoms. After three to four weeks of consistent input, the patient was able to have drinks via sips and eat a normal diet, although she did experience ongoing hesitancy when eating and still preferred softer options.

The patient being motivated to complete relaxation exercises and her next of kin and nursing team being keen to support with specific relaxation cues during mealtimes were key to successful outcomes regarding her eating and drinking. They were also verbally communicating at the sentence level, with significantly improved dysfluency symptoms, although these were ongoing at the point of discharge. I have since regularly worked with patients with FND and continue to find relaxation helpful for communication and swallow input. Distraction techniques have also been helpful to reduce dysfluency symptoms.

Although there have been many positive experiences with FND, there have also been quite a few challenges. A particular challenge tends to be the negative stigma attached to this diagnosis. This can, in turn, lead to challenges around patient flow and discharge planning within the acute hospital setting. I've had patients on my caseload who experience swallowing and/or communication difficulties and would benefit from a full multidisciplinary team input but have often felt pressured into immediately 'fixing' these issues or supporting discharge home despite the patient experiencing ongoing issues. This leads to challenging conversations within the multidisciplinary team, especially on acute stroke wards, where patients are often discharged home quickly or are waiting for a transfer to a medical bed, which can take some time and thus impact bed availability for hyperacute stroke patients. Overcoming this challenge is difficult but is eased by the multidisciplinary team developing a better understanding of each other's roles with this caseload. As the negative stigma seems to be challenged, patients with FND do seem to be getting more time in an inpatient setting for much-needed immediate input than they may have historically had. Though there are ongoing challenges, there does seem to be a gradual shift in multidisciplinary team working and management, which is reflected in recent multidisciplinary team discussions relating to the lack of a recognized patient pathway for this cohort and enthusiasm to develop this.

Of course, another significant challenge is not having any education on this condition at university and since FND being on my caseload is not uncommon, I do feel quite strongly that teaching on this disorder at universities should be included. Initially, I felt inadequate and doubted myself as a therapist when working with FND, due to a lack of experience and knowledge.

Through research, joint working with senior colleagues, joining an informal UK-wide supervision group, and understanding multidisciplinary team roles, my confidence in case history gathering, assessment, and treatment is starting to increase. The case history gathering, and subsequent input, is quite different from my usual neurology-based caseload. This is mostly due to the psychology and trust-based nuances that are often ingrained in FND, but I enjoy the difference in approach and have developed a great interest in the field. Despite the challenges of the variable effects of treatment, multidisciplinary team management, lack of funding and pathways, I have grown to genuinely enjoy working with, and advocating for, patients with this condition.

62

A Detour to a Better Place

Female, 37 years old, US

FUNCTIONAL MOVEMENT DISORDER

I am a patient with FND and a healthcare provider. I was diagnosed after going to many doctors and having many tests, just like many patients with FND do. Even though I was working in healthcare at the time, I had not heard of the term FND. I had heard of conversion disorder, but no one mentioned that terminology. I had no frame of reference or context that I would be diagnosed with FND. I had no idea that my own profession would be the one that would help me recover and reach a new normal.

My background is somewhat complex. I have experienced many medical challenges since I was a child, but none of them stopped me from having a regular life, an education, independence and a career. I was in my early thirties when I woke up one day and didn't feel right, with difficulty using my left arm and leg. Due to my history, I just shrugged it off as maybe I was getting sick and just needed to rest. It became apparent the next day that something wasn't right when I continued to have weakness on the left side. I started the process of seeing many doctors, and a long journey to a diagnosis.

I continued working despite the movement disorder I had developed. It took about nine months before I was diagnosed. I did have to stop working about eight months after the symptoms developed. When the patients you are working with are asking if you are okay, it becomes almost impossible for them to trust you as their provider. Being in healthcare did not exclude me from having some disheartening experiences with medical professionals, as many patients with FND have had. You might think there would have been some different level of empathy and compassion, but honestly there was not. I waited about five months to get into the programme that did help me improve. During the time I had to wait to get help, I did what most nerdy scientific-minded professionals do: I started researching the diagnosis and treatment. Due to my profession, I was able to grasp the concepts of the potential for recovery. I tried to work on things on my own and had some small improvements, but I quickly realized I was going to need someone to help me.

One week of treatment was all it took for me to get back on the right path. Most patients need more and formal follow-up, but I was able to continue my own rehabilitation independently. I was able to return to work one year from the date I had stopped working. I have continued to work full time for the last five years. There has been more than one relapse, but they were short-lived, and I was able to use all the tools I gained from rehabilitation to quickly improve.

I believe I will always have FND. My goal is to just keep it under the threshold so none of the outwardly recognizable symptoms come out. There are still the invisible symptoms, but I am mostly able to keep them under control as well. I have to put the work in every day, but the payoff is worth it. I am able to do what I love. As hard and debilitating as FND can be, for me, my life is better overall because of the experiences I went through. I never take anything for granted. I am grateful for all the simple things in life. I live my life to serve others, which I have recognized as my purpose since I was young. I understand that my story and my circumstances are unique to me, just like everyone's are unique to them. I don't want to diminish the challenges that people face with this diagnosis. There is such a large spectrum of symptoms, presentations and personal circumstances that affect potential recovery.

These are the keys I believe helped me in recovery: I did not let the diagnosis of FND define me or limit my expectations of my life. I had a purpose for my life that I had believed in since I was in fifth grade, and I didn't want anything to stop me from fulfilling that purpose, even if my life would have to shift in a different direction. I believed in my heart that I was going to get better. Instead of looking at FND as a roadblock to my life, I looked at it as a detour to a better place than I could have ever imagined on my own. I was blessed with an amazing family and supportive friends. I have grown up with a strong spiritual life that has helped me through the most difficult times.

You can see that none of the above have anything to do with formal treatment. Although that was important in my recovery, I believe the other pieces are what helped me over the top. I hope my story can give hope to others that there is potential to live a productive and fulfilling life with FND.

63

FND and the Psychiatrist

Liaison psychiatrist, 20 years' experience
of working with FND, UK

Discussing the psychological aspects of onset or persistence of
FND is harder than it should be.

I have worked as a psychiatrist with an interest in FND for
20 years – 15 of them as a consultant in a large teaching hospital. In
my clinical practice, I have been interested in the personal context
within which symptoms develop – my influences being time spent
gaining experience in family therapy, training in interpersonal
psychotherapy, and undertaking research using standardized
interview methods (originated by the group in Bedford College,
UK) for eliciting events and difficulties that can precede the onset
of illness.

What I learned, and research shows, is that the majority of
people with FND have indeed experienced some sort of adult life
problem in the time leading up to onset. It is rarely 'traumatic',
usually taking the form of an intractable predicament or dilemma
in personal relationships or the immediate social world. In her
books, neurologist Suzanne O'Sullivan (2015, 2021) highlights
individual (sporadic) cases she has seen in the clinic and the mass
(epidemic) cases she has studied for professional interest, and I find
the lessons she draws from these are familiar from my own rather
different clinical background.

One of the functions of psychiatry in the management of

FND is to explore the origins of the disorder and consider, with the patient, how an understanding of personal and social circumstances can be built into a plan for recovery. How does the encounter go? A few people are (perhaps surprisingly) already comfortable with the idea and have come to a similar conclusion themselves. Many are bemused – the idea of psychological factors leading to onset or persistence of physical illness seems odd and not immediately in line with their personal experience. A minority are hostile, perhaps angry: no doubt a commoner response than a psychiatrist sees in clinic because it is likely to have led to refusal to accept referral, but not a universal response.

Patients express scepticism or rejection of psychological factors in a number of ways. A common early riposte is based on a misunderstanding – that what is being proposed is that the illness is imagined or made up. It is linked to a frequent complaint about not being believed: I see this response as a reflection of a wider cultural lack of recognition of psychological factors in physical illness. Related is the complaint that psychological formulations are a cloak for medical ignorance, or that they indicate unwillingness to take certain states or certain people (women for example) seriously. A lack of immediately obvious traumatic experiences can make the need for further exploration seem forced and a common belief, even among clinicians, is that 'normal' people don't get psychologically caused illness so it can't be relevant in previously well-functioning individuals.

Towards the end of her book about FND, Suzanne O'Sullivan asks: 'If psychosomatic symptoms are so ubiquitous, why are we so ill-equipped to deal with them?' (2015, p.283). I have a number of candidate answers to that question. One is that, faced with negative or sceptical responses to even raising the possibility, most clinicians have little idea what to do next. Lack of understanding of the nature of psychological and social influences on illness is explained by their near-complete absence from the medical curriculum at undergraduate or postgraduate level. Nobody really discusses these things in Freudian terms anymore and everything important can't be called 'trauma', but unfamiliarity with more up-to-date approaches makes it difficult to have a satisfactory conversation with a questioning patient. Poorly handled referral to a mental health professional can easily sound dismissive or evasive and in truth there are few specialists available to whom referral is possible. One corollary is lack of awareness of the range of therapeutic approaches that might be helpful; cognitive behavioural therapy is not a panacea.

More research, both explanatory and interventional, would help. Here are some personal thoughts about what needs to change in the meantime about how we approach FND. They relate just to this one aspect of the clinical problem, which is how to become better at discussing and responding to the possibility of life problems as relevant in onset or persistence of symptoms.

First, we need to challenge the idea that psychological formulation is demeaning and misguided. Illness is a state of symptoms and associated disability, and it is nonetheless real for not being associated with abnormality in bodily organs. Disagreement about the cause of illness is not the same as disbelief in the reality of the illness. In this respect, I find some writing about FND is unhelpful. Saying 'it's not all in your head' is meaningless at a literal level, and hints implicitly at agreement with the idea that psychological explanation is dismissive. Emphasizing the history of Freudian thinking about 'hysteria' – often in any case misrepresented – before going on to talk about brain function or hardware/software metaphors has the same function.

Clinical practice would benefit from early introduction of the possibility of psychological influences and treatments, and not just in relation to co-morbidity or response to chronic illness. Further psychological exploration and treatment when appropriate should be offered to all, and especially encouraged in those who do not recover completely with standard rehabilitation approaches. Of course, to achieve this we need to develop more services able to offer therapy integrated with physical rehabilitation services, and support a wider range of interpersonally oriented approaches.

Clinical education at undergraduate and postgraduate levels needs to improve greatly. Illness with normal investigations features too little and too late in most curricula; the nature of psychological and social influences on health and how adversity of all sorts can be meaningfully related to illness is hardly taught in most schools. And finally, clinical skills in discussing these matters with patients are picked up (or not) on the job when they should be taught and developed at every stage in training and practice.

References

O'Sullivan, S. (2015). *It's All In Your Head*. London: Vintage.
O'Sullivan, S. (2021). *The Sleeping Beauties*. London: Picador.

64

The Importance of Language in FND Treatment

Clinical psychologist, three years'
experience of working with FND, UK

I've worked with patients experiencing FNDs prior to, during, and since my professional training in clinical psychology. I feel the need to say that I did not intend for my path to look this way, but I am thankful that it did. I was drawn to neuropsychology early in my career. I had the fortune of being a psychology assistant in stroke rehabilitation. I was regularly asked to see patients with functional stroke symptoms. Although always willing to try, I was never quite sure how best to help these patients. I remember feeling incompetent and under-supervised. Where appropriate, I would offer mind-body links to explain the influence of stress and trauma on the body. For some patients, this helped; many others seemed to be alienated by this suggestion. To my surprise, being transparent about the unknowns of FND was often appreciated.

Most confidently, I think the patients valued being listened to. This can be in short supply in busy hospital settings. Patients with FND often have complicated lives and histories; being able to bear witness to their story, should they feel able to share it, can be a powerful experience for narrator and listener. To listen without judgement and unconditionally believe someone's experience may not sound like a big ask, yet I fear for patients with FND it is rarely provided. What's worse, I fear that many patients with FND are harmed by the dismissive and pejorative messages sent by the very professionals whose role it is to help.

My key learning from this role was recognizing how important language can be. The words we ascribe to patients can shape our views and distort our judgements. Terms commonly used in healthcare discourse around patients with FND can be pejorative, ambiguous and blaming. Commonly observed terms have included 'pseudo', 'psychosomatic', 'malingering', and (my personal pet hate) 'behavioural'. These terms have no place in good healthcare for anyone, certainly not for people experiencing FND.

We also ought to be aware of the harmful ways in which ward narratives can develop in response to an FND diagnosis. Following a negative MRI scan, Mrs P in bed six is suddenly 'the functional patient', 'not a real stroke', 'pulling the wool', or even 'bed blocking'. Remember, all systems have the potential to become punitive, dismissive and corrupt; believing that you are exempt by merely 'being a healthcare clinician' is an effective way to confirm you are guilty and complicit. Discourse and language can be hard to alter, much harder when we do not try. It shames me to think how much more I might have done.

During, and since my clinical training, I have been working in a service that specializes in treating individuals with functional seizures. Unfortunately, services such as these are rare, and what provisions do exist are limited and hard to access. Even those patients I can see will have to first wait two years on a waiting list to start treatment, following what will have already been a lengthy process to receive the diagnosis. I often feel privileged about my role but dissatisfied by the limited availability of treatment. I cannot think of a patient group more deserving.

At the eventual point of being seen by my service, many patients are understandably desperate for the treatment to work. Expecting treatment to work is important, and fortunately it often does; but that constant pressure within the first appointment has always weighed heavy on me. Many of those who attend the first appointment want to be anywhere but seeing a psychologist. Patients can be sceptical, resistant and even angry – an understandable set of responses to being thrust into a treatment that may not fit their understanding of their symptoms. For these patients, instilling belief and hope that psychological treatment could be relevant and effective is half the battle, although at times a difficult one. Being honest and persuasive about the expectations of treatment, while not alienating the individual, and adhering to ethical integrity is often the first real task of treatment. At the end of the first appointment, it can feel rewarding to know I have given this my all; yet this still fails to protect me from the shame and self-doubt if they do not come back for the second.

65

Listening to My Body

Female, 38 years old, UK

FND INCLUDING FUNCTIONAL
SPEECH DISORDER

I suddenly acquired FND three years ago. I came home after a family day trip out with my children and suddenly had whole body paralysis with pins and needles everywhere. I couldn't move. I couldn't talk. The immediate diagnosis, and later an inpatient rehabilitation stay, gave me a false sense of security: the professionals know what this is, know what they're doing and how to fix it.

The limb movements and my strength returned quickly, but my voice did not. The pins and needles moved around my body and varied in intensity. The doctors were confident the voice would return at some point as there was no structural reason for it not to. It was just a matter of when, but they had no advice on how to achieve that. I had never heard of FND when I acquired it, so I naively believed that, once my voice had come back, it would be the end of it. Friends and family around me stayed optimistic, following my lead of immediate acceptance and positivity as a way to cope.

After rehabilitation and still with no voice, I was referred to a speech therapist. I didn't speak for a total of five months. My family already knew a small amount of sign language so I could still communicate, or I typed out notes on my phone. I became very insular and felt alienated in groups of people, although it came with a certain amount of relief that I didn't have to contribute or interact with others if I didn't want to. As time went on, I became less accepting and more confused and frustrated about what was happening. I wanted answers.

By the time the referral to the speech therapist came through, I could talk in a whisper with a stammer. The therapist didn't directly teach me to talk fluently again because in her words, it 'would be pointless'. I knew how to talk, and no amount of willingness or exercises would cause my speech to return clearly if it didn't want to. Instead, we focused on getting my body into a relaxed and calm state, we practised deep breathing and really noticing what was going on inside my body rather than my thinking mind. We delved into my subconscious and tried to work out what it was that my body and self needed.

Due to my past experiences, I had developed some pretty strong and painful core beliefs about my sense of self and worth. I had learned from a very young age to ignore my body and numb my feelings and emotions, that my internal experiences were wrong or incorrect. My needs were less than everyone else's, and I did what I was 'supposed' to do. I had some pretty strong conditional values imprinted on me and I was trying to live up to the high Western standards of what it is to be a woman and a mother. We came to realize how intensely I had learned to ignore my needs and put myself last. On the flip side, it meant I was determined, I worked hard, I showed up, I achieved and was 'successful'.

The FND part of me was shouting loud and clear that fundamentally something wasn't okay and I couldn't ignore it any longer. My way of life and thought patterns were not sustainable. Subconsciously, those core beliefs, that something about myself was wrong, had come to the forefront. I had reached a point where I was too scared to talk or move; I was living in a permanent 'freeze' state. My body was telling me in a really crude way that I had to listen to it and not to my thinking mind.

I am living in a continual fight, flight, freeze, flop state, aware of potential threats all the time. My threshold for threat is very, very low. I now see the FND as a completely normal way for a body to work and it doesn't necessarily need 'fixing' by medical professionals; it's just not currently socially accepted or usually visible in the general population. There is nothing wrong with my mechanism of response: some people might feel sick or get sweaty palms if feeling anxious, I can't talk.

My symptoms are still present and fluctuate in severity and length. It helps me to view all the symptoms (including the newly acquired ones) as temporary, I just don't know how long the temporary bit is. I don't try to actively change them otherwise it perpetuates feeling stressed out and they last longer. I have confidence that my body will sort itself out eventually, when it is ready.

I am making progress with learning to recognize and challenge some of my core beliefs and expectations. I still ignore or forget how to look after myself, so I actually need the FND symptoms as a reminder to come back to a more relaxed state of being. I don't have the skills to fully recognize my internal or emotional state yet, so the FND does it for me. When life becomes difficult, the severity of my symptoms is a pretty good gauge for how heightened my nervous system is.

I use a variety of ways to calm my body and mind, anything from playing or listening to music, reading, yoga, meditating, colouring, cooking, sewing, or avoiding technology for a few days. I know this is what I need to do, but I'm only human. I have responsibilities and can be distracted by more enticing activities. I've had to come to accept that I can't actually do it all.

Alongside trying to be in a more relaxed state, I've found the biggest help has been learning self-compassion skills. Being non-judgementally aware and talking kindly to myself has really helped me come to terms with what has happened. It's difficult for someone who wants to know the answers to have a disorder that isn't really understood. My FND is an ironic reminder that my entire body and being exists, not just my head.

66

An Emotional Rollercoaster

Husband of person diagnosed with FND, UK

I think I would characterize my journey as a partner of someone who has FND as an emotional rollercoaster. It's an experience which has made me learn about myself and is challenging in many ways.

For me, the initial episode which led to my wife's FND diagnosis was an extremely worrying time. During this first episode, she had near total paralysis and loss of speech, so she was unable to communicate anything about what was going on. While we were waiting for the ambulance, all I could think was that she had had a stroke. Although the paramedic and ambulance crew reassured us that they didn't think it was a stroke, it was still clear something very serious had happened. The diagnosis of FND was actually made pretty quickly, which started to give me some hope, as I thought that, as there was nothing structurally wrong with her brain, a full recovery was possible. The fact that she recovered her ability to walk and write again over the next two days seemed to support what I was hoping for, although she still could not speak.

I feel fortunate that my wife was quickly offered the choice of an inpatient stay of several weeks, to have intensive therapies and support. This was obviously a practical challenge, given we have three children (not to mention the impending Covid-19 lockdown, which we didn't yet know about!), but seemed to be a real step towards recovery. I think my wife found the stay in hospital beneficial overall; for me, it proved something of a reality check as we saw people with quite serious long-term symptoms from their FND, and the clinical team were realistic about the variable prognosis and timescale.

In a strange way, coming back home during the first Covid-19 lockdown worked out well. We had time and space as a family to try and start adjusting to my wife's FND symptoms. At this point, she was unable to speak, and it remained so for months, which was sometimes frustrating on both sides but generally manageable. More concerning were the frequent seizures and limb paralysis, especially as they seemed to come on without warning. I hated seeing my wife have seizures and saw the impact of the after-effects, so I wanted to do anything I could to stop them from happening. As I would guess many people do, I began to look for patterns of what I thought triggered symptoms, such as when the children were fighting or being loud. My wife tried to tell me that the FND was too complex and random to find such associations; however, I think in an attempt to make some sense of the situation or feel like I had some control, I continued to focus on what seemed to me like stressful situations and put a huge effort into avoiding them.

Ultimately, the stress of trying to make sure the home environment was 'trigger free' was negatively affecting my mental health and making family life unpleasant. I was so concerned about putting my wife first and trying to meet her needs that I was not looking after myself. I would have long periods of 'holding it together' followed by an acute episode of anger or depression. Finally, realizing this was not a sustainable way of living, I have had counselling, CBT, and I have been prescribed antidepressants as part of a long process of acceptance of her FND and the impact it continues to have on our life, and my powerlessness to change much of this – a process which is not yet finished. I still get frustrated and annoyed with FND, particularly when my wife's symptoms are bad and there is high demand on my time to give practical support, or I have to stop what I am doing and go to help her. It can feel as if I have to be ever alert and ready to help out.

However, to end on something more positive, the FND

diagnosis has not changed the person underneath. My wife still makes me laugh more than anyone else can; she is a great mother to our children, adapting what she can and can't do with them, and still active in the community, albeit in a modified way. There are challenges, but overall life is getting better.

67

A Long Diagnostic Journey

Female, 33 years old, UK

FUNCTIONAL SENSORY DIFFICULTIES

I have sensory FND, which includes numbness, tingling, headaches, fatigue and weakness. I was diagnosed earlier this year but have been experiencing FND for six years. I've seen so many inspiring and remarkable FND stories, but I couldn't relate to any of them as their symptoms weren't like mine – invisible and difficult to diagnose. Admittedly, sensory FND doesn't make a compelling online video, so I'm hoping I can connect with you through writing. Here's my story.

How it happened

I was in a yoga class six years ago and we were about to do a backbend, plow pose, where you put your feet over the back of your head and take on the form of a badly crafted Swiss roll. Before going into the posture, the teacher warned us not to turn our necks as it could lead to a nasty injury. So, we were in these postures and the teacher walked around the class checking our positioning. She was at the other end of the room to where I was and she said something to the class – now, when someone talks to me, I tend to look at them. So, I turned my neck to the left and turned it back just as quickly, thinking 'Oh no, I wasn't supposed to do that', and thought nothing more of it.

After the class I noticed a tingling in my fingers and toes. I went to A&E and a (rather irked, understandably) doctor gave me anti-inflammatories and sent me home. The tablets helped but didn't deal with the problem entirely. It was like stretching an elastic band that doesn't quite go back into place once the tension is released.

Going steady – for a while

Whatever the condition was, it remained stable for around four years. It caused discomfort, but it was never prohibitive. I cycled every day, went for a long run at the weekend, climbed and figure skated, all the while experiencing this inconvenience. I'd tried getting help for it, seeking every specialist I could think of – chiropractor, physiotherapist, neurologist. It worsened incrementally after cycling 54 miles and falling off a climbing wall – but even then, no real concern from doctors. Once you have enough evidence pointing to your symptoms being in your head, you wholeheartedly believe it. After all, there weren't any visible outward symptoms.

Until two years ago that is. It was 3am and my flatmates and I were in a bay at the hospital. I'd already asked why we were in the hospital 16 times, but it was the final time that my short-term memory – and the realization – stuck. I'd had a seizure. Part of the treatment following your first seizure is a discussion with a neurologist. Until then, I was given the standard set of restrictions: no cycling, swimming, driving, booze [alcohol] or baths. But I did gain the proof of a physical symptom. Someone might actually believe there was something wrong with me!

This was around six weeks before the first Covid-19 lockdown and the extra restrictions that came with it. I'd tried making up for the lack of exercise by walking more but I was finding myself feeling dizzy and experiencing sensitivity to light. I hardly went outside during the first lockdown (frankly, I was at greater risk of developing deep vein thrombosis than catching Covid), and I noticed my symptoms improve. That cemented the belief that exercise made me feel worse, as it had done to some degree in the four years beforehand.

Over time, it was taking less and less activity to bring about intense pins and needles, headaches, neck pain, muscle weakness and fatigue. All still invisible. Well, except for a rash and red-hot itchiness that would come about when I hadn't taken my pain medication. I haven't seen it in any other FND cases.

The diagnosis

The neurologist I spoke to post-seizure wasn't able to help much. It wasn't until two neurologists, and a new GP, an osteopath, several diagnostic tests and over two years later that I got a diagnosis of FND over the phone. He spent a lot of time explaining evolution and how I'm more anxious because I'm primed to care for babies and that makes me more predisposed to FND. I found it difficult to take this seriously as I don't want children. Then he gave me links to a couple of educational websites and told me to do 15 minutes of mindfulness a day. That's difficult to do when, for six years, you've believed your house is on fire and when it's confirmed that it is, you're told not to panic. But you can't help but panic because your house is on fire.

I came away from that conversation feeling adrift, with so many questions: Is this progressive? Is it reversible? Is it a disability? If so, where can I find support?

I was at work when I took the call. After getting through the second half of the day, I bought a tray of nuggets and went to bed bawling, believing that I was on my way to a wheelchair.

226

How are things now?

It wasn't until I did a university questionnaire on FND diagnosis that I realized how many treatment options there are. I had to speak to someone else to get more information on this condition.

I found an amazing clinic and was seen by a neurologist and a neuropsychiatrist. The appointment lasted around two hours; they were thorough and patient and showed the concern I'd been seeking for the best part of a decade. Not only did they confirm the diagnosis, but they assured me it wouldn't get worse and could really improve with a combined treatment of physiotherapy and psychotherapy.

I'm awaiting physiotherapy and I can't wait to start. By this time next year, I might be back on my dusty neglected bike while wearing a pair of heels and experiencing the tingle of exhilaration – not the tingle of sensory FND.

68

Breaking Down the Barriers

Neuro-physiotherapist/cognitive
behavioural therapist, 30 years' experience
of working with FND, UK

'I want a therapist who knows what they are talking about.'

I trained and specialized initially as a neurological physiotherapist working with long-term conditions. Although this specialism was a great foundation and skill, I still felt I was missing something in order to help some patients diagnosed with FND to achieve a better quality of life and unblock some barriers to recovery:

'This feels very scary and easier to withdraw/avoid.' 'If I get better, how will I cope with anxious things?' 'I have flashbacks of the event.'

It has been a wonderful learning journey to find optimal skills as a physiotherapist to help people diagnosed with FND. I will continue this journey throughout my life. However, to date I would like to share what training I have found that has improved my skills. Patients want to be listened to in a very skilful way – a way that does not bring about judgement in any shape or form, a way they can trust and be open to, to reveal the barriers to recovery and then be able to treat collaboratively and effectively.

'Why do clinicians not listen or actually hear me?' 'I feel judged as if I am not believed.' 'I want to work with my therapist rather than be told what to do. I want to do therapy in my way and terms and pace.'

With all that in mind, I then trained in CBT to a master's level. This opened a whole new approach to dealing with some of the challenges not only for my patients but for how I saw things as well. We all know everyone is different and people react or behave the way they do for very good reasons. The training helped me to understand coping mechanisms, safety behaviours, emotions, anxiety and how the body reacts to thoughts and behaviours. It teaches self-management in a very supportive way.

'I know why I am the way I am and it's not my fault.'

Physiotherapy and CBT intertwine the physical with the psycho-logical in a non-threatening way to bring about change. They help to understand perhaps the more complex blocks to recovery. Let's keep working together and learn in order to bring about the change the patient wants.

69

An FND/Functional Seizure Focus Group: Experiences of Invalidation and Therapy

Trainee clinical psychologist, consultant neuropsychologist and consultant neuropsychologist, UK

To try to fill the gap locally (i.e., no funded services), we conducted a pilot project offering six sessions of psychological therapy (psychoeducation and grounding techniques) for individuals with a diagnosis of NEAD (functional seizures) or FND. The outcomes were evaluated as part of a trainee clinical psychology service evaluation project, which included an online focus group, attended by four people.

We wanted to assess service user satisfaction, to find out what was and was not helpful about our therapy, and ask people what an ideal service would look like. During the focus group, insights about people's journey through services were shared, as were interesting ideas about what such a service could seek to achieve.

Experiences of services

The group described a difficult journey through services. Learning that their experiences were a collection of symptoms that were part of a recognized neurological/psychological condition was a relief. A theme throughout the meeting was that participants felt invalidated and unaccommodated by healthcare services, with the exception of the pilot psychological intervention that they had received from our service. It was shocking and sad for us to hear the group's stories about how their condition had been managed by professionals and services. For most, it was the first time their experience of FND/NEAD had felt validated by a healthcare professional. All of the participants offered anecdotes about being treated dismissively or inappropriately by professionals:

> She [healthcare professional] told me it was all in my head and the reason that it was all in my head was because I was overweight, and I've got no friends. If I lost weight and got friends, it would all go away, and I'd be perfectly fine.

It was appalling to hear how the group were blamed by some professionals for their condition.

Also described were experiences of being invalidated during other routine appointments (e.g., with their GP, cardiologist). The group agreed that being given a name for their condition had been helpful, rather than stigmatizing, as it enabled them to navigate services more effectively. Furthermore, it allowed participants to share its name with family and friends, which led to a sense that their difficulties were being taken seriously.

Participants described being offered interventions in the past that they didn't feel targeted their needs; for example, being prescribed medication for epilepsy or pain. They contrasted this with the psychological intervention, which was instrumental in helping some of the participants to begin the process of acceptance. One person reflected, 'I learned that it's an actual condition... It's not just in my head. It's not made-up.' Furthermore, they felt that the

therapy intervention helped in recognizing triggers and interven-
ing earlier to reduce symptoms.

An ideal service

The group agreed that there would be great value in an FND/
NEAD psychology service, which wasn't surprising to us. All participants agreed that the most important part of such a service would
be offering teaching to other professionals in other services. This
was surprising to us in that, this was felt to be more important
than being offered individual therapy. This spoke to the pivotal
importance, from our patients' perspectives, of addressing negative
attitudes and experiences of invalidation across the healthcare
system for people diagnosed with FND/NEAD and being treated
with respect as service users.

Participants reported that experiences in other services, where
they had felt stigmatized and misunderstood, were so traumatizing
and shaming that effort towards reducing such experiences should
be prioritized. It was frustrating to hear about instances in which
participants had NEAD attacks/FND episodes in public. Emergency services were alerted, and they were brought to A&E against
their will and waited a long time for tests such as an ECG which
they knew were not going to yield any useful information and
weren't an appropriate use of resources. One participant described
being pulled to their feet by staff and ordered to 'walk it off'. They
reported feeling misunderstood when they tried to explain this to
professionals and felt that this could be avoided if there was greater
awareness of NEAD/FND by emergency personnel. Participants
shared how angry their treatment by services had left them and
we, the facilitators, shared this sense of injustice.

Participants reflected that they would also benefit from further
therapy. All participants agreed that a six-session course of therapy
was insufficient to meet their needs. Along with more one-on-one
therapy, participants shared that support groups for both individuals, and also their family members, would be helpful: 'It might

be something that may help us if we were all able to be with other people with the same condition and discuss the bad stories but also the good things and what works.' This was interesting to us as there seemed to be a desire to build a supportive community around the condition.

Within an ideal service, an initial medication assessment, a course of therapy and regular reviews coordinated by a doctor and therapist were suggested. One participant explained:

> People who have got cancer or other things. I know it's a horrible disease, but then they get more check-ups. So why don't we deserve check-ups and not just chucking medication at us? I don't know why I am on [medication] half the stuff I'm on.

This appointment would function to review their use of coping skills, along with the benefits and side effects of prescribed medication.

Reflection

Although we were familiar with the often-negative experiences of people with FND/NEAD in their attempts to access support from services, hearing individual's sharing stories about this brought home the isolation this population experiences. The focus group gave space for creative user-led ideas about how to build better services for individuals with FND/NEAD, but also how this could operate more widely, beyond offering individual therapy. It was heartening to hear the group's positive experiences of psychology and the sense that their difficulties were finally being seen by professionals. 'She was ever so lovely, and she got me [understood me]... It's like making that bond with someone as well. I'll never forget it.'

70

Being 'Normal'

Neurologist, 25 years' experience
of working with FND, UK

Being normal is not very fashionable these days. There is no normal. We should celebrate diversity, including neurodiversity. 'Psychodiversity' is not a word – probably because of stigma – but if it was, I think we should celebrate that as well.

But 'normal' hangs around all of us, as something we crave to varying degrees, and it especially hangs around in the clinic, as something we reach for to help ourselves and our patients. Let's look at some examples:

- 'That's okay, everyone gets some white dots on their brain scan as they get older, what you have is NORMAL for your age.'
- 'You do have a lot of back pain, but the MRI of your spine is NORMAL for your age. Around 50 per cent of people your age would have a disc bulge like that, and actually they really don't correlate well with current or future back pain, so we don't need to worry about it.'
- Patient with FND: 'As well as my previous symptoms, I'm having these times when one half of my face scrunches up and I get double vision. It's really horrible and scary'. Doctor replying after examination: 'You've got some functional

facial spasm and convergent spasm; that's NORMAL for FND.'

- 'I know it really worries you that you go in another room and forget why you're there. But about one in three young people in their twenties do that every week - so to some extent, it is NORMAL.'
- 'I wish I was just NORMAL again.'

I'm interested in normal, because as a health professional it seems like something we are incredibly bad at studying. In fact, I'm not really a 'health' professional - I'm an 'illness' professional trained to find things that are abnormal, dysfunctional and broken in the body.

At no stage in my training did anyone tell me what normal health is. There is an assumption that to be healthy is to be symptom free, physically and mentally active and free to do whatever your income and time allows you to.

But actually, that is not NORMAL, that is a description of an unusually SUPERNORMAL state of health which is only achieved by a small proportion of people most of the time.

In reality, NORMAL is all kinds of bad things that we would rather not have. National surveys of symptoms and health show that on average we feel tired 'some of the time'. Studies of cognition show that not only are we walking upstairs and forgetting why we are there, but we also put our keys in the fridge, lose our cars in the car park, forget the names of someone we know well and forget a really important item from the supermarket. On average, NORMAL is feeling pain in our back and knees from time to time. It's normal to have headaches from time to time. Only a tiny percentage of the population never have a headache in their life. When I lecture students on headache, I ask who has never had a headache and point out that the few who put their hands up are, statistically anyway, the abnormal ones. We all feel dizzy sometimes, we often can't sleep or sleep too much, the list goes on. And we have other kinds of not normal. We might feel unusually sad, or suddenly anxious - perhaps for perfectly good reasons, but perhaps sometimes not. We might have a slight tendency to be obsessively compulsive, getting addicted to a mobile phone game, or want to check the lock a few times.

How are we supposed to know whether we are healthy if we don't know what normal is? Shouldn't they teach this stuff at school?

It was my ambition, at one time, to write an A–Z of normal – maybe even a popular book called 'NORMAL'. But, useful as that might seem at one level, I would worry now that it would be seen as 'anti-diversity' which would be counterproductive.

What has all of this got to do with FND? Well, quite a lot, I think.

There are many people out there who have transient or mild neurological symptoms which are clinically 'functional', but they don't have a disorder. Mostly they seem to want an explanation but not be told they have a disorder. Some really hope that what has been happening is in the realms of NORMAL.

People with FND often get into a tangle, with health professionals doing tests and presenting results to them without proper reference to NORMAL. 'You have wear and tear, and a bulging disc' is a very different message to 'You have normal age-related change that is unlikely to be relevant to your pain.' This kind of medical harm is unfortunately very common and people with FND understandably latch on to test findings that are normal or probably normal which can get in the way of self-management of FND.

I meet many people who were in the SUPERNORMAL category before they became ill with FND – 'always on the go', 'the life and soul', and 'such a bubbly personality'. They did three separate jobs, looked after their kids, other people's kids, their mother, baked cakes for the school fete and had time to go to the gym and run half marathons. When a supernormal person becomes ill unexpectedly, especially with something as frightening and poorly managed as FND, then is it reasonable for them to expect a recovery back to being supernormal? Often as a health professional I'm encouraging them to return to a state of being NORMAL, like the rest of us.

How can I do that if they (or I) don't clearly articulate what that looks like? I never want to hear the phrase 'new normal' again after living through the Covid-19 pandemic – but it is a new normal that is often required. Sometimes the old normal was, with hindsight, unsustainable, or possibly even one of the reasons why FND happened in the first place. The new normal may be living with FND as a long-term condition.

So, a plea to allow the study and appreciation of NORMAL, while acknowledging that we are all unique and diverse and the last thing we want is a society where everyone is the same.

Helpful Resources

We hope that the stories in this book will enable readers to learn more about FND. At the very least, the many stories we have collected from around the world show how many lives are affected by FND.

In addition to the many strategies that contributors have described throughout the book, and which have helped them to deal with their FND, we thought readers might find it useful for us to include a guide to further resources. We appreciate that websites or videos cannot replace the direct contact with a clinician or therapist, but they may enable people to improve their understanding of the difficulties they face and to find their own solutions. We are also aware that no list we could provide would be complete or completely up-to-date. The amount of information available about FND is increasing rapidly.

The resources listed below should be relevant to individuals with FND, people supporting someone with FND informally or professionally, and those wanting to know more about the condition – in other words, everyone.

Importantly, the editors of this book live in the UK or US. We realize that most of these resources may be most relevant to one sub-group of people with FND, namely those who speak English and have access to listed websites and publications.

FND patient-led organizations and services

FND Hope is an international organization specifically for individuals with FND. There are separate organizations in the UK, Netherlands, Canada, Australia, US and an international service: https://fndhope.org

FND Action is an organization based in the UK: www.fndaction.org.uk

FND Dimensions is an organization based in the UK: www.fnd-dimensions.org

FND friends is an organization based in the UK: https://fndfriends.com

FND Australia Support Service Inc. is an organization based in Australia: www.fndaus.org.au

FND Matters NI is an organization based in Northern Ireland: https://fndmattersni.org.uk

FND together is a charity based in Canada https://fndtogether.com

FND health professional-led organizations and services

The FND society is an international society for healthcare professionals and researchers in FND, but which community members can also join. It holds conferences, hosts webinars and aims to promote research and education in FND: www.fndsociety.org

Neurosymptoms FND guide is a multilingual online guide and app on all things related to FND started by Prof Jon Stone, one of the editors of this book in 2009: https://neurosymptoms.org

MyFND is an app designed to help people with their FND symptoms started by Dr Chris Symeon in London: https://myfnd.co.uk

FND Australia is a network of health professionals interested in FND in Australia and has information for patients and families as well: https://fndaustralia.com.au

AIDiNEf is the Italian Association of FND and is a joint health professional and patient organization promoting awareness and support for people with FND in Italy: https://aidinef.it

ag-fns.de is a German network of health professionals dedicated to improving research and services for people with FND: https://ag-fns.de

Functionele Bewegingsstoornissen is a website in Dutch with detailed self-help information about functional movement disorders: https://functionelebewegingsstoornissen.nl

Information specifically about functional seizures

Information on all things related to functional seizures:

- www.nonepilepticattacks.info
- www.nonepilepticseizures.com

Dis-sociated, a documentary on functional seizures: www.youtube.com/watch?v=MA1EYAg9y5k

Two books on the treatment of functional seizures and other functional disorders in children and adolescents:

- Savage, B. *et al.* (2022). *Treatment of Functional Seizures in Children and Adolescents: A Mind-Body Manual for Health Professionals.* Samford, Queensland: Australian Academic

Press. This book can also be accessed via the following URL: www.australianacademicpress.com.au/books/details/346/ Treatment_of_Functional_Seizures_in_Children_and_ Adolescents_A_Mind-Body_Manual_for_Health_ Professionals

- Kozlowska, K., Scher, S. & Helgeland, H. (2020). *Functional Somatic Symptoms in Children and Adolescents: A Stress-System Approach to Assessment and Treatment*. New York, NY: Palgrave Macmillan. This book can also be accessed via the following URL: https://link.springer.com/ book/10.1007/978-3-030-46184-3

Information for young people and families living with functional seizures: www.neurokid.co.uk

A free graphic novel telling the story of someone with functional seizures called *Not There*: https://neurosymptoms.org/en/media/ other-media/not-there-a-graphic-novel-about-functional-seizures

If you want to read more personal and professional experiences of functional seizures:

- Reuber, M., Rawlings, G.H. & Schachter, S.C. (2020). *Non-Epileptic Seizures in Our Experience: Accounts of Health Care Professionals*. New York, NY: Oxford University Press.
- Reuber, M., Rawlings, G.H. & Schachter, S. C. (2018). *In Our Words: Personal Accounts of Living with Non-Epileptic Seizures*. New York, NY: Oxford University Press.

FND advocates

While there are many FND advocates, we wanted to highlight two in particular:

- https://fndportal.org

- https://fndrecovery.com

Services for FND

You can find a map of providers with an interest in FND through FND Hope's provider map: https://fndhope.org/living-fnd/managing-fnd-find-provider

A list of FND specialist centres in the UK can be accessed via FND Action: www.fndaction.org.uk/specialist-care

We also recommend that you speak to a healthcare professional in your country for information about available treatments.

Services for people in distress

If you are in severe distress, having a crisis or in an emergency, please contact the relevant services in your country. For example, in the UK this may be 999 or your local mental health crisis services.

We have included a link below that takes you to a directory of international mental health helplines. This helpfully organizes services via countries and what difficulties each service can support you with: www.helpguide.org/find-help.htm

About the Editors

Dr Gregg H. Rawlings is a clinical psychologist and lecturer at the University of Sheffield. He completed his PhD from the University of Sheffield, investigating the experiences of living with functional seizures.

Professor Markus Reuber is Professor of Clinical Neurology at the University of Sheffield and an honorary consultant at the Sheffield Teaching Hospitals NHS Foundation Trust. He is Editor-in-Chief of *Seizure - European Journal of Epilepsy*.

Professor Jon Stone is Professor of Neurology at the University of Edinburgh and a consultant neurologist with NHS Lothian. He has run neurosymptoms.org, a self-help website for FND, since 2009, and is the first secretary and co-founder of the new international FND society (www.fndsociety.org).

Maxanne McCormick practiced as a paediatric physician assistant until 2009, when debilitating symptoms from FND forced her to resign. She runs the blog www.FNDrecovery.com, and in 2020 she was a speaker for the FND Hope virtual conference. She is based in Monument, CO, USA.

Index